THE MIRROR INSIDE:

A JOURNEY TO FINDING ANSWERS TO ULCERATIVE COLITIS FROM WITHIN

ZOE CHLOE DOUGLAS

ISBN-13:978-0692244012
ISBN-10:0692244018

DEDICATION

Dedicated to the wonderful you.

TABLE OF CONTENTS

CHAPTER 1

DOWN TO THE ROOTS: EXPLORING THE PAST TO UNDERSTAND THE PRESENT

I'm a 38-year-old woman who has lived with Ulcerative Colitis for the last ten years. It is not easy to talk about my life. And although I know there are many women and men in the world who battle this disease every day of their life and have faced many struggles similar to those I have faced, it doesn't make my telling you this any easier.

At the end of the day, you realize it doesn't matter how many people have fought the same battle, your battle is yours alone to fight and hence unique. Each of us copes differently. The questions may be the same, but the answers are most often different. What helps is sharing these different experiences, helping others know what to expect, how to prepare. Most importantly, know that it is possible to lead a better quality of life, no matter what you have had to live through already; that only hope and positive action can fight the two sisters known as Fear and Grief.

I was less than four years old when I met Fear. Like a

dark stain, it would spread steadily inside my stomach every time I watched my parents fight. I was too young to know why my father beat my mother. I only knew the unpleasant and uneasy feeling of fear and disgust I would feel deep down in my stomach and the unsettling flutter I would feel in my heart. I remember many incidents after which I'd see my mother badly bruised and battered. There were times when I would not be able to keep away and I'd rush to help my mother or would try to get help from others. At such times, not only would I get hurt in the process, but my efforts to get help would prove futile as well. East German society in those days was not very forthcoming in matters of domestic violence.

Fortunately, my mother divorced when I was about five years old and I never saw my father again.

It was many years later that I realized Fear and Grief are ugly sisters who not only impact your life but also your health. And even though after the age of five, I never had to see my mother abused again, Fear and Grief, along with suppression, visited in other forms and I found the fabric of my childhood and youth to be deeply stained. It is this realization that has led to both the question and answer to my Ulcerative Colitis.

I was born in a small town in the state of Thuringia in what was known then as the German Democratic Republic (GDR) or more commonly, East Germany. My mother was a kindergarten teacher. We were not well-off, but we had everything we needed. No one in those days lived lavishly in a socialist country. Most people didn't even have a phone in their home. If you wanted to make a call, you had to go out to find a public phone.

It's hard for most who grew up in capitalist Western countries to imagine this life. People led incredibly frugal and controlled lives. As if there was a shortage of life itself. From a very young age, you were trained to hold back and be sparing with everything, whether it was food, money, things in the house, your thoughts and ideas or even love. You expressed less. You consumed less. You imagined less. You felt less.

My mother was an embodiment of this in many ways. I knew she loved my brother and I, even though I was also very aware that she never quite expressed this love fully or openly. She worked very hard to provide for us and perhaps, given the circumstances she was raised in, she did the best as she could.

I remember how we didn't always get even basic fruits, like oranges and bananas. We would get them only once a year and had to stand in a line to get the rationed amount: a few per person in each family. I can still remember standing behind a long line of people, on a chilly winter's day, waiting to get my hands on a bag of oranges. We'd take the fruit home and my mother would divide everything equally between my brother and I. Whether it was a simple fruit like a banana or a "luxury" commodity like a car, everything was painstakingly rationed and, in some cases, had to be ordered years in advance. If my mother wanted me to have a car when I turned eighteen, she would have had to request one when I was born.

Our lives were policed and controlled in other ways as well. There were only a few state-run channels available on the television. So exposure to the outside world was almost non-existent. But we lived close to the border and sometimes we'd catch a radio or TV station from West Germany. We had to watch these secretly, so even the neighbors would not know. The state encouraged citizens to report on each other to the Stasi in case they found someone undermining the Communist government's rules or principles.

The Stasi was one of the most hated and feared institutions of the East German Communist government. It was developed from the internal security and police divisions established in Soviet-occupied Germany after World War II, but members' roles and responsibilities were not clearly outlined. Broadly speaking, they were in charge of both domestic and foreign threats that would challenge the Communist state. Thuringia's close proximity to West Germany meant that it was always on the front lines of the Cold War and monitored more vigilantly by the Stasi.

Many may find this picture of a Communist state to be cliché, but having lived in one I know just how real it was. Every child, from the age of six to fourteen, had to be part of the Young Pioneers, a concept similar to Scouts in Western nations, but organized with the objective of indoctrinating every child with the socialist ideology and preparing them to become members of the Freie Deutsche Jugend (the Free German Youth), the official Communist youth movement. With the extensive influence of the erstwhile Russia Federation over East Germany, learning Russian language was also obligatory.

For children, the controlled environment began at school. Teachers were often rude and harsh. Regular dental check-ups were mandatory at school, but the dentist was not required to get permission from parents before treating their children. So often were treatments unnecessary and performed without anesthesia. When I look back now, I find it was an insane practice to just decide and conduct treatments without informing or taking consent from parents.

In school, we were trained to know what you can talk about and what you cannot. I remember being constantly mindful to not speak of certain things for fear that the teachers may report me to the Stasi. It was a fairly repressive time to grow up. It often felt as though I could not have my own voice and opinion and instead had to obey and do things even if I didn't agree with them. As a result, I grew up to be shy and suppressed.

I was fourteen when the Berlin Wall came down, but it took a while to break free from the intensive indoctrination of more than two generations. From my perspective, these early years of suppression and conditioning played a vital role in my health and my approach to life.

Sometimes, when I reflect on my childhood in East Germany, and try to recall what my aspirations were, I'm hard-pressed to find even one. I assume it is because we were so isolated from the rest of the world and suppressed that we weren't allowed to imagine our own futures. Perhaps a symptom of being raised in a Communist state is that a person grows up without much of a mind of their own or a free spirit.

It has taken years for me to break free from this state of being, in more ways than one. I'm aware that this suppression and tendency towards submission lead to many bad choices and decisions in my adult life.

Even at home, our lives were quite emotionless. My mother, as I said earlier, never quite displayed her love and affection in an obvious manner. Most often, she would go through the motions of being a mother devoid of feeling. I think she felt a greater sense of responsibility than attachment, which drove her to look after us. Even my relationship with my brother was cordial but distant.

I'm not sure whether it is because I was deprived of these emotions in childhood and then again in later relationships, but ironically, I find myself today a loving, compassionate and gentle person. Sometimes, I think I am a bit too compassionate, putting my own needs last. This is another aspect I have realized about myself in my journey in dealing with Ulcerative Colitis.

But one of the most significant things I have learned to help me understand how to treat my Ulcerative Colitis is this: oppression and suppression of any kind has a definitive and long-term impact on our health. The earlier we realize this, the closer we are to getting better.

You can see this clearly when you think about how obsessive control, whether wielded by the state, your husband, your parent or your boss, brings you down, makes you feel cornered, overwhelmed, helpless and trapped. It increases your vulnerability and diminishes your ability to make decisions that will lead you away from the situation that's bringing you down. In fact, when you make decisions in a vulnerable and "cornered" state, you invariably land up in a worse situation. Sometimes, we dig ourselves deeper and deeper into it, and begin to believe that we don't deserve any better.

CHAPTER 2

PUT A LID ON IT: SOCIAL, POLITICAL, AND RELATIONAL SUPPRESSION AND THE IMPACT IT HAS ON HEALTH

Throughout the world's political history, we know that when states target, discriminate and oppress a group of people over a period of time, that group starts to internalize the oppression. Simply said, we start to believe what we are told and see ourselves that way. Women who are in abusive relationships will say, "I probably deserved it." Persecuted minorities will say, "It's true, we don't belong here, this isn't our country/state." In feudal societies, you find farmers saying, "This is what we are meant to be" or "We are beneath those who are educated or wealthier than us."

A small example: one socially accepted view is that girls are not good at math. If you think about it, most women will "naturally" think that we are not innately good at math. We're surprised when we see a girl win a math competition. As women, we've basically internalized a stereotype that is meant to put us down.

There are many sociologists who believe that when people from a suppressed society internalize myths, misinformation and have quelled their natural instinct to think for themselves for years, it makes them feel that in some way they are inherently not as worthy, capable, beautiful or good. In essence, you turn the experience of suppression inwards. You behave according to the stereotype and you wholeheartedly believe that it is true.

I find this a common occurrence among women, people who come from poor families and people who have faced political and social suppression.

There is an ongoing discussion among health professionals, alternative therapists, psychologists and sociologists about the direct link between years of suppression (emotional and otherwise) and a person's health. I'm aware of this now, but I didn't initially when I was trying to understand my disease.

I can reflect now on my childhood and recall the oft-repeated message that emotions or being overemotional is a bad thing; that it was a sign of weakness and showed that you were not in control. As children, we got accustomed to denying and hiding our emotions to the extent that it became a habit. However, today I've come to realize that denying the existence of our emotions is like denying our awareness of our selves. Awareness of who we are and what we truly want influences how our minds function and how our bodies react.

A friend's grandmother once told me, "You know why women live longer than men? Because we can cry." The simple act of crying relieves stress and calms one down but many of us feel even that is something to be ashamed of.

To rephrase the words of Thomas Scheff, Professor Emeritus, UCSB, over years we learn to suppress what we feel and think and we build a backlog of emotions like fear, anger and embarrassment. The more emotions pile up, the more overwhelmed with life we feel and the more intimidating the prospect of feeling and expressing emotion becomes.

It's a vicious cycle. Suppressing emotions and thoughts not only leads to discontent and ill health but also violence. In their book titled, *Emotions and Violence*, Thomas Scheff and Suzanne Retzinger explore the theory of the emotional causes of violence. They propose in the theory that shame is the primary or the ultimate cause of violence; especially shame held in secret. Scheff says, in his essay in their book, "When a person is intensely ashamed of being ashamed, they hide their shame by covering it with anger and aggression." He goes on to also include withdrawal, depression and silence as alternative results, but points out that often domestic abuse has a direct correlation with these secret emotions.

Psychologists believe that people, particularly suppressed and emotionally deprived women, are often attracted to those with similar issues. However, the suppression of emotions plays out differently between men and women. Experience leads me to believe Scheff's theory: men compensate for their suppression of emotions with violence, while long-term suppression leads women to internalize the idea that they aren't good enough. It's an awful situation to find yourself in. You look for love and kindness even though in your heart you believe you don't deserve it, while your partner thinks physical or psychological abuse will give him better control over his life and situation.

The ability to be aware of what is going on inside you, to understand what your body is trying to communicate, to think for yourself and to not be bullied by stereotypes, relationships, doctors or a state is critical to achieving a healthier and happier life and to making better choices and decisions about your life.

It took me years to truly realize this. I can say that

perhaps if I didn't have Ulcerative Colitis, I may never have been forced to find my way out. Over the initial years of being in and out of hospitals, I noticed a direct correlation between my stress level and UC flare-ups. Clearly, abuse and emotional strains during my relationships were making it worse. It wasn't a dramatic morning, a singular moment of realization, or an epiphany - as with most of life's lessons, I very slowly, little by little, came to the conclusion that I must end the sources of stress if I wanted to lead a better life. No longer would I put my happiness in the hands of others to control.

I decided I would not allow others to suppress me nor would I suppress myself. This was the start of a journey to understanding my body, my Ulcerative Colitis and to ultimately find the solutions to better manage my life.

CHAPTER 3

THE INITIAL YEARS

I was 28 years old when one day I discovered a little blood in the toilet. I didn't pay much attention at first. Perhaps I wanted to avoid confronting a problem looming over head. I had enough issues already. It had only been two years since I had moved from Germany to the United States. Settling in a new country and culture and getting your bearings is challenging enough. But I had wanted to grow personally and professionally and so, by the time I turned 26, I had taught myself to speak English. We never learned English in school, but I started learning the language when I was 23. I had worked hard and saved enough to start a new life in a new country, and although the future was uncertain I was self-reliant and hardy enough to know that I could make it.

In this new phase of life and in a new country, I met a man who I found to be very loving and caring, at least at first. You could say that I was dazzled by how indulgent he was and how much attention he gave me. When you're a girl who has grown up in a fairly cold and reserved society and you come to a country where people are far more free and expressive, you may be swept off your feet more easily. We got married, but the honeymoon phase didn't last very long. I think as soon as they know they have you, men often drop their effort and increasingly take you for granted. Other things begin to emerge, too: control, resentment, anger and power struggles. People can't hide who they essentially are and what they truly want forever.

Soon the unpleasantness in my marriage spilled over into my professional life and I found it to be a big challenge to manage both. Also, my husband resented me working, so I decided not to work to keep the peace. But the domestic abuse and psychological trauma didn't end. It never does. The sacrifices and the changes you make in your life to accommodate your partner's demands are not unlike the medication that you take for UC. They only provide temporary relief, when the entire objective is to address and remediate the symptoms, not necessarily find a cure or eradicate the problem. I think we approach so many of life's struggles in the exact way doctors approach UC; we are unable to understand how to cure it, we avoid making the difficult decisions, so we try to patch things up with Band-Aids the best way we know how. Not one of these bandages is a long-term solution and after short remissions, we invariably have flare-ups.

Once again in my life, I felt cornered, overwhelmed and suffocated. I was unable to see my way out and unable to see how the stressful situation I was in affected my body. And then my body spoke. It indicated in no uncertain terms the stress it was enduring and the impact of that stress. The blood in my stools and the frequency of the diarrhea over the next few weeks become worse and worse. At first I ignored the problem. I guess I didn't want to face any more trouble.

I saw my fear grow daily, from a mild sense of concern to the point where I was too afraid to even want to know what was wrong. I didn't go see a doctor until two months later when I realized that I was spending more time every day in the bathroom than outside it. I had grown extremely weak and was finding it hard to do even the smallest chores in the house. I didn't understand what was happening to my body and when I finally went to see a doctor, I had to go through a series of tests before I could get a straight answer.

I remember the day I was told that I had Ulcerative Colitis and I would have to take medication for the rest of my life. I remember the tears welling up and rolling down my face. Despite all of my life's struggles, I had never actually been seriously ill. I had never taken any medication. All of a sudden, the prospect of having to take medication for the rest of my life was shocking and unimaginable. They told me there was no cure. What they didn't tell me is how much it would change my life. What it would entail, what I should expect or what I must do. When I think about it now, the approach of simply treating the symptoms was a defeatist attitude. It's like they are telling you: "There's nothing really you can do. Just put a Band-Aid on it." The medical system doesn't realize that certain chronic diseases that impact a person's life in a very public and private way have to be addressed in a manner that is more thought out. For most patients, it's difficult to initially understand what is happening to their body and how it will affect the rest of their life. It is a chronic illness that you are made extremely aware of every day and has the potential to take over your entire life.

The day I was diagnosed, the doctor told me of a support group I could join for patients with Ulcerative Colitis. At that time it was too early; I was still partly in denial of the disease and much too stubborn. I didn't want to get involved in groups where all you hear is intense talk about UC and Crohn's disease; it was bad enough to have been diagnosed with it. I didn't want my disease to be my entire reality. I didn't want to live and breathe it every moment. I didn't want to hear or talk about it. I already would have to make adjustments to my life to accommodate it and I didn't want to be drowned in other people's battles with UC as well.

I also believe there is quite a bit of brainwashing in these support groups. This belief was confirmed some years after my diagnosis when I finally attended a meeting and was immediately put off by all the pro-surgery talk. There were those who had already had their colon removed and were eager to talk about how successful and wonderful it was. There were others who were about to make that choice and perhaps were zealously convincing themselves as much as others that they had made the right decision. There was a lady who jokingly bragged that she no longer needed toilet paper. I'm afraid I found little to laugh about. It was depressing just being there. And when she mentioned how the bag accidentally came off once, I had to stop myself from running out of the room.

I have never quite believed in the power of support groups. I can say that at least with regards to UC. I think there are many others who also find it more depressing than empowering. I came to realize early on that we must discover our own sources of knowledge and support.

The day I was diagnosed with UC, I remember returning home from the doctor in a daze. I told my husband and while he initially tried to understand the situation, over the subsequent weeks it was clear that I couldn't expect any more from him. In fact, what made the whole situation worse was that the domestic abuse and unpleasantness continued. And for many years I tolerated it all with the hope that he would change, but he didn't. I continued the marriage, battling interpersonal issues as well as my health issues. It wasn't until many years later that I finally decided to get a divorce.

Soon after I was diagnosed, I happened to have applied for training and qualification to work in the real estate business. But my condition worsened and I had to put my training on hold. I was too weak and couldn't sit in a classroom or be out in public because of constantly having to get to the toilet.

Within months, my weight plummeted from 145 lbs to 110. For the greater part of the following years, I was bed-ridden and hospitalized. I couldn't leave the toilet; anything I ate went right through. It was the hardest time of my life. I felt miserable and sorry for myself when I saw others my age enjoying their youth, a great family life, friends and work while I was undergoing so much pain and most of the time lay completely debilitated.

I started to withdraw from friends and family. It is not a disease you can talk about openly. It is extremely personal and, having grown up in a society where we didn't share emotions freely, I found it difficult to share. But I knew my mother and friends were deeply worried about me.

Before the onset of UC, I enjoyed meeting friends, going out, working and exercising; I led a fairly actively life. Although I didn't do so much socializing after marriage, I was never a frail weakling. It is not a picture I had ever imagined for myself. Now, after many months of living with UC, I was reduced to exactly that. Somewhere, such a realization plays a great deal on your mind. Your physical debilitation makes you more vulnerable and ashamed. You don't want to have to depend on others, and yet you find yourself increasingly in the position of being more dependent. You feel publicly embarrassed by the disease itself.

There's also that sense that you're doing nothing. You feel your body is not the only thing that is wasting away, your mind and your life is too. This is one of the first battles you have and until you can find peace with your body, you continue to fight it. It takes some time to learn that you're not wasting away; you're actually just giving your body and mind some much-needed rest. You have to tell yourself that there is nothing to be ashamed of or feel guilty about. Many of us grow up in families or communities that believe you should just knuckle up and get on with it. Throughout my childhood, I never saw my mother show any weakness, despite the grief from her marriage and taking responsibility for us from a young age. She worked multiple jobs, worked hard and long hours to give my brother and I a good upbringing. I never saw her dependent on anyone, no matter what. I never saw a moment of weakness or vulnerability in her. So initially, one of the greatest battles I fought was feeling guilty about being sick and wasting space and myself. It only put more pressure on me, increasing my stress and making my UC worse. But with time, and as I became more spiritual, I was able to cut myself some slack and be at greater peace with my body as well as my disease. In fact, spirituality and its role in helping me gain better control and longer remission is something I will discuss further in another chapter. It taught me to question my tendency to be judgmental and, in particular, why I was judgmental of myself to such an extent. I asked myself if being guilty or ashamed was helping me become better at something. Was it helping with my situation? Was it helping anyone else? Clearly, it wasn't. That's when I realized I needed to stop and take a moment to soul search.

In these initial years of dealing with UC, I had a really hard time managing the disease. Doctors didn't tell me how I could reduce the chances of flare-ups, they didn't advise me about food. In fact, they said UC has nothing to do with food, so I could eat whatever I wanted. This is so far from the truth. Food has a lot to do with flare-ups, as I later would realize. This ill advice was perhaps indicative of the larger issues with our overall health care system. It's far more profitable to have a patient keep coming back for treatment of the flare-ups than to give them a holistic solution so they can sustain their remissions. However, I would never say I've had bad doctors, only that the system isn't engineered to have doctors look beyond simply suppressing the symptoms when they appear. Even today, UC is not given the same consideration as there are so many other life-threatening and life-altering diseases that have proper support structures.

One of the first things a UC patient suffers is a phobia of food. Look at how we react when we simply have a mild case of food poisoning. The first thing we'll say is, "Oh God, I don't even want to <u>look</u> at food."

Just imagine this feeling, but amplified – that is what a UC patient feels. You don't just get this feeling for a short while or in passing. You begin to feel it all the time, it takes over your life and wherever you go; when you look at food, you think of the toilet. In fact, eating becomes associated with the fear of abdominal pain even before you've finished your meal.

The frequent spells of diarrhea that accompany UC can cause such a strong sense of humiliation that social isolation and low self-esteem starts to set in. UC takes a serious toll on your work, your family and your social life. In fact, surveys suggest that almost half of patients complain of being completely incapacitated for at least 180 days of the year.

I think for me, in the beginning, it was more than that. The disease's progression was slow, but it grew very deeply. It was the hardest time of my life. If I wasn't in the hospital, I was in the emergency room. As with most chronic conditions, my immune system began to fail. I was going to the toilet 17 to 20 times in a span of just 24 hours. I was losing a lot of blood, so much so that I ended up getting a total of twelve blood transfusions over a period of three weeks.

I remember my first transfusion being the hardest to accept. I was scared and fought with the idea for 16 hours, not wanting to get the transfusion. But the doctors declared that my situation was life threatening and my hemoglobin was so low (only 4.2g, which should be between 12 and 16) and my blood pressure so high that I wouldn't make it to the next day without a blood transfusion.

I suffered from extreme anemia, excruciating abdominal pain, chronic diarrhea, poor circulation, chronic fatigue, edema in my legs and ankles, arthritis, insomnia, hair loss, receding gums, an irregular heartbeat, a blood clot in the brain, declining vision, heavy night sweats and chills all at the same time.

At one point I was unable to bend my knees and I wasn't able to walk or lift anything. There was a point when I was so frail that if I wanted to drink water I couldn't even lift up a normal cup or glass, only a light plastic cup.

I changed doctors several times, hoping each time that the new one would be able to treat me differently or offer a new solution. But they all put me on more or less the same medications. As my condition worsened, the drugs prescribed to me were more severe as were their side effects. My illness didn't respond very well to conventional medication. Once again, I feel therein lies another failure of our medical system. It doesn't take into account those who don't respond well to the drugs offered. It doesn't provide us with an alternative other than surgery.

I was put on Asacol, Remicade, Rowasa, Canasa, Priobiotics, Flagil, Cipro, 6-MP (Mercaptopurine) and blood thinners, the last of which was given to dissolve the blood clot in my brain. At one point, I was given the steroids Hydrocortisone and Prednisone for eleven days straight – the former was given intravenously and the latter was given orally. These are only a few of what I tried; the entire list of medications could fill several pages. I even saw alternative medical practitioners, but nothing helped. During one of my hospital stays, I remember, I was so badly off that I had a daily visit from a Pastor who sat next to me and prayed. I never had anyone pray for me before.

And although I must have seen more than a dozen doctors from the start of this disease, there is only one particular doctor who had grown to care deeply for me. She cared so much that when they found the blood clot in my brain, she began to fear that I would not actually make it. One day, I found her standing next to my bed with tears welling up in her eyes.

In those early years, my UC was out of control and I spent weeks at a time in the hospital. Doctors told me that I had one of the most severe cases of UC they had ever seen. During one of these stays, I remember a time when I was put on an IV and I had to go to the toilet. I decided to take the IV pole and walk. It wasn't far, but I was so weak that I couldn't go fast enough. I bled all over the floor. I was so embarrassed that I started cleaning up the floor with one arm while the other was still attached to the IV. I didn't want the nurses to see the mess I'd made. This is what I mean when I say you have to be prepared to not punish yourself with shame and guilt because you are sick and none of this is deliberate.

While in the hospital, I was given a PICC line and was fed, or nourished I should say, with TPN through an IV.

A PICC line is used when a UC patient can no longer digest food or when the ulcers in the colon are so widespread and severe that doctors don't want any food to pass through at all. The PICC line delivers what is known as Parenteral Nutrition. It's also called Total Parenteral Nutrition (TPN) when it's the only source of food for the patient. The food is in the form of a liquid and consists of a very precise mix of nutrients, making it safe to pass straight into your veins. The PICC line is inserted into a large vein that won't be irritated with PN. You can stay on a PICC line for months, although in my case I only had to be on it for a few days.

In the third week of one of my many hospital stays, I was put on an intravenous immunosuppressant to stop the bleeding. It had to be given every few weeks and had fairly severe known side effects, like lupus and a higher risk of infection. Lupus is a chronic inflammatory disease where your body's immune system attacks its own tissues and organs. Inflammation caused by lupus can affect many different parts of the body including your joints, skin, kidneys, blood cells, brain, heart and lungs. Although the drug worked at first, I ultimately developed antibodies against it and was no longer able to receive the drug.

In the meantime, prolonged and high exposure to Hydrocortisone and Prednisone had started to deplete my bones' density so much so that a year after the treatment I began to complain of hip pain. When I went to get a DEXA Scan that measures bone density, the technician asked how old I was. When I replied, he was aghast and said my bones were far too thin for my age, then asked had I ever been treated with steroids.

No longer able to work or go out with friends, my primary and constant concern was to be close to a toilet at all times. If I went outside the house, it was hard to relax and not think about it. These initial years with UC were therefore extremely lonely. When I reflect back on it now, I wish I had better guidance; that I was stronger within and didn't feel so guilty or so diminished. When you are already vulnerable and then something awful like this happens to you, you tend to fall harder and deeper into darkness. Bringing yourself out takes longer, greater effort and faith in yourself and in God.

CHAPTER 4

STRESS AND SPIRITUALISM

One of the primary reasons for writing this book is that I'd like to tell readers and others who suffer from UC that I strongly believe my Ulcerative Colitis was induced by stress. I have no doubt that stress also causes my flare-ups. Although you'll find over a hundred articles on the Internet that disprove this and your doctors will tell you that they have found no empirical proof of a connection between stress and Ulcerative Colitis, I believe there is a vast chasm between what doctors know about UC and what patients experience.

My knowledge on the subject is based entirely on my own personal observations and trial and error.

Even those who don't have any form of IBD or IBS can get an upset stomach when they are stressed or nervous. For example, you feel queasy when you are upset, afraid or have sense of foreboding. Most negative emotions are linked to your gut. "Deep down" is where you hold the most intimate of emotions. It is also what you use to measure how you feel about a situation.

Even those who don't have IBD will have more frequent bowel movements or diarrhea when under stress. In my personal journey of adjusting to UC, I have come to observe that if I watch how my body reacts to stress and what causes it I can better manage my UC proactively and avoid flare-ups.

One of the first things is to learn to recognize what causes you and your body stress. Most often, by the time we recognize stress, we are already so deep in a situation that already has had an adverse impact on our body. When I was young, I would get headaches due to stress. I didn't know what caused it at the time; all I knew was that I'd get jaw-breaking headaches that would encircle my head like a crown of pain. Each time I'd get one, it would take hours to subside.

Our body responds differently to varied levels of stress. For pre-historic man, stress or anxiety would give him either the adrenalin rush he needed to face a hungry tiger or it would give him the speed to run in the opposite direction. In fact, it is this natural "fight or flight" response of the body that makes the digestive system slow down so the body can free up energy to fight or run.

In modern times, while situations may be less life-threatening, they are more intense and they originate from multiple sources. We could be facing stress because of the workload we have, a difficult boss or colleague, the demands of our jobs, financial commitments, relationships, family and more. Each of these factors presents stress in varying manner and degrees and our body responds differently to each one.

For example, if you have a performance evaluation at work, you might get a headache; in more severe situations, you might feel nauseated or get an upset stomach. There are those for whom higher levels or prolonged periods of stress bring on issues of hair loss, high blood pressure, diabetes and heart disease. Stress has both short-term and long-term impacts on our body. Short-term impacts are those we can easily observe and quickly correct.

We often think of stress only in terms of mental strains, but physical strains have an impact, too. Obesity puts an inordinate amount of stress on your body. Your body may react to this kind of stress in a different way than someone else's body would. Often people with obesity issues have knee problems. Certain drugs and medications induce physical strains that can cause irreparable damage to the body.

Eating certain foods like high-fiber vegetables or dairy products can stress the digestive system of some UC patients.

It is therefore important to understand stress – both mental and physical - and the impact it has on your health. This helps you to eliminate its source, maintain your remission and make the right decisions for your treatments and your life.

One of the easiest ways to recognize stress is to break down the stages of your body's response to it. Try to observe what happens when you are stressed and how your body reacts as that stress worsens. This is an exercise in "listening to your body" and, as a UC patient, it is a tool that you will most often rely on.

For example, I know I'm stressed out by something when I have a headache. Depending on the intensity of stress I feel, my body's response varies from the queasy sensation in my stomach to irregular and heavier breathing, tension in my jaw, insomnia, etc.

Being a UC patient, I've explored extensively what stress can do to my body, how to recognize its signs and how to cope with it. Each of these signs is also a sign of other health issues, so it's important to rule those out and confirm that what you are experiencing is actually stress-related and not something worse. Once you know that it is stress-related, you should resolve it before it transforms into a full-blown UC flare-up. Some of these symptoms have very basic and simple solutions, although that doesn't mean they are not effective or that you should take them lightly. For example, if you're having sleepless nights, don't have coffee after 3 p.m. Or, if you have sore muscles, take a hot bath with Epsom salts. If you're feeling overwhelmed, talk a walk in fresh air, you could also take yoga classes. The latter is something I have found really helpful in unwinding. Sometimes the simplest solutions save us from bigger problems.

Headaches are one of the simplest ways for our bodies to tell us it's under stress. Stress headaches in particular are characterized by their tight crown-like manifestation. One of the ways I've learned to deal with this is to use a simple breathing exercise practiced in yoga. You sit in a quiet place, it could be a room or in a quiet area of the park. Sit up straight, straighten your shoulders, rest one arm on your knee and use the other to close and free the right nostril. Gently close the right nostril and inhale slowly through the left. Lift your finger off the right nostril and slowly exhale. Do this for about five to six minutes. During the exercise, you essentially focus on your breathing by inhaling slowly from one nostril and exhaling slowly from the other. The technique is called Chandra Bheda in yoga and helps to quiet the mind and cool the body. In yoga, it's believed that each nostril plays a role in the body's overall balance – while inhaling from the left and exhaling from the right cools the body, the reverse warms up the body.

There are several other breathing techniques in yoga that can help relieve stress from the mind as well as body, but they need to be learned from an experienced instructor. Always remember to give the instructor your complete health history so he can suggest the right techniques for your body.

Another common sign of stress is lower back and neck pain. These are centers in the body where muscles contract and spasm when the body and mind are under attack. When back pain is caused by mental stress, it's known as a psychosomatic pain. The terminology doesn't mean the pain is imagined, rather it implies that there is an actual physical manifestation of something psychological. Stress-related back pain is also known as Tension Myositis Syndrome. TMS is examined with a multi-dimensional approach. Physically, a doctor will determine if your back or neck muscles have become weak, if nerves are getting pressed or irritated. Emotionally, you'll need to understand if you are suffering from anxiety, anger or depression. Psychologists also believe exploring the cognitive aspect: whether you have negative thoughts, are pessimistic or feeling hopelessness. Environmental aspects of TMS could include a bad marriage, loss of a job or financial problems. Based upon which of these are causing the TMS, your doctor will suggest a treatment course. Physical factors can be treated with physiotherapy and pain medication. Emotional factors are treated with appropriate medication, e.g., muscle relaxants and anti-depressants. Learning techniques for managing psychological pain and biofeedback helps when treating emotional and cognitive factors. Of course, environmental factors are worked through with counseling or psychotherapy.

There are people for whom stress may not bring a distinct lower back pain or neck pain but a more general soreness in the body. Just like with the back muscles, other muscles contract as well in response to stress, increasing the production of lactic acid and leading to pain. It helps to take a warm bath with Epsom salts so the body can rid itself of lactic acid in the muscles. When you take a warm bath, the brain releases endorphins that also help with pain relief.

Insomnia or sleepless nights is another common sign of stress. Whenever I get these, I take action quickly, because sleeplessness puts a strain on your digestive system, causing your stomach to release acids into the lining where there's no food to digest. I've observed that taking a magnesium supplement before going to bed helps. Use a relaxation technique from yoga to help lull your body to sleep.

Frequent spells of the flu and falling ill can also be a sign that you are under severe stress. High levels of stress hormones reduce the efficiency of the immune system, leaving you more vulnerable to viruses and bacteria. In a study at Carnegie Mellon University, researchers surveyed a random group of volunteers about what was going on in their lives and then infected them with a cold virus. They found that men and women coping with stress, ranging from a bad marriage to unemployment, were twice as likely to get sick as those with fewer problems. The same study also found an increased resistance to cortisol in the participants, a stress hormone that keeps the body's inflammatory response to infection in check. Taking some time off, even if it means just a weekend away, helps greatly. Or if you can't get away, then set aside part of your day to do something that you find fun and interesting. Engaging your mind in a positive way helps with dealing with short spells of stress and maintaining longer stress-free periods.

Sometimes, it helps to delegate tasks, reduce your load of responsibilities and not feel guilty about it. If going out or socializing is putting pressure on you, don't do it!

It's important to learn how to relax in general when you suffer from Ulcerative Colitis. Find out what helps you calm down when you're very anxious or feeling pressured. It might be something as basic as taking a walk by yourself, reading a book, doing a breathing exercise, having a cup of green tea or taking a nap. Make a list of these things; writing them down helps you to internalize the solutions.

Reduce stress for yourself on a daily basis. As I said earlier, if socializing is causing stress, take it easy. While it's good to socialize for your own quality of life, it's also okay to sometimes say no. If you go out with friends out of obligation, it defeats the purpose of being out with friends.

At work, go to meetings fully prepared and a few minutes early. Find out before you go where the toilets are and don't eat anything that might have an adverse impact on you. This way, you can work with complete ease and you have resolved all the usual possible points of stress.

Here are some of the ways to cope with stress on a daily basis:

Have a positive attitude: I know this sounds preachy and easier said than done, but thinking good thoughts is essential to coping with a life-long illness and even life's general challenges. If at first you can't find positivity, simply think of things that bring a smile to your face – even if it means just reading a joke. Or spend a little time in doing something that you are good at and take great pride in. It could be something as simple as baking a cake or doing a bit of gardening. These are things that bring an element of positivity and lead you eventually to having hope in the future and faith in yourself.

Learn to let go: Don't drown yourself with ownership at the workplace and at home. Learn to delegate. Learn to not get too bothered when things don't turn out the way they ideally should. Don't beat yourself up trying to either take on all responsibilities or trying to finish everything you start. How successfully you can let go depends on how well you prioritize your life. Prioritizing what is important to you helps you distinguish and focus on only that which is essential to you, so your energies are not spread thin over a large variety of things.

Push the envelope: Challenge yourself every once in a while. It encourages you to feel like you can take on anything. It gives you a sense of achievement, self-confidence and self-worth. Go for a hike or run a race. Exercising certainly helps at so many levels. It'll help in relieving stress, building self-confidence, leading a healthier life.

Carve out "me time:" It could be a hobby, meditation, a walk; whatever you choose to do, it's important to spend some time alone. We often expect others to live harmoniously with us, even though we don't know how to live with ourselves. Spending time and doing something alone helps you understand yourself better. It's a time when you can indulge yourself and grow as an individual. It also makes it easier to be okay with putting yourself first. Carving out some "me time" is the first step towards putting yourself first.

In case you are unable to do this on your own, it is perfectly fine to seek outside help. Unchecked stress and anxiety can build up and if it's aggravating your UC symptoms and keeping you from leading a better life, it is perfectly fine to seek help.

For example, I have found that it is extremely calming to talk to my Pastor, especially during the dark periods of long hospitalization and severe flare-ups. I know many who find guidance from psychologists and counselors help them get better control over contributors of stress.

No matter whom you seek help from, it's important to have faith in yourself. Aim to get to the point when you think that you can actually reduce your stress and manage UC; the point where you can prevent becoming overwhelmed by the disease and by stress in general. I know I personally have many sources of anxiety and it's taken me years to train myself to mitigate them down to a more manageable state. In fact, I know women who have children, pets, homes and careers to manage alongside their UC, who could say, "What could you know about stress?" But it's not a competition. Every man and woman has his or her own significant contributors of stress, and while finding the time to identify these properly and then listing ways you can reduce their impact may seem unreal and unachievable, believe me, when you're facing a severe health crisis, you realize you have to find the time. You have to put yourself first and you just have to learn to not feel guilty about it. I told myself that I'm no good to myself or anybody else unless I stay strong and know how to look after myself.

It was perhaps one of the hardest things I've ever had to do - learn to put my own needs first and not feel guilty about it. And the best part is that it's not like I've turned into a selfish person. My friends and family have realized that I have re-prioritized my life and they are happier for it. My friendships are stronger, my work is better and I have great clarity about what I expect from a partner and do not intend to repeat past mistakes. Being able to look after yourself and control your contributors of stress makes you feel a strong sense of empowerment.

Looking within yourself for solutions as well as support from others is something spirituality and religion have taught me.

CHAPTER 5

SPIRITUALITY

I can never forget the day when I was finally allowed to walk in the hospital garden to get some fresh air after having spent almost three weeks inside. I remember just standing there for a few minutes, breathing, filling my lungs with fresh air like I had been hungry for it for years, and at the same time feeling as if I were doing it for the first time. I was fully aware of every distinct element: the smell of fresh grass, the coolness of the air, the cleansing feeling one gets when one breathes fresh air. I felt aware and was thankful for this awareness.

I had never been a believer before I fell ill with Ulcerative Colitis and even then, it was a slow and very gradual process. Prior to knowing I had Ulcerative Colitis, I think I took life mostly for granted. I believed that everything I had in life was normal and expected and there was nothing extraordinary about it. In my mind, nothing evoked or warranted any appreciation. But somewhere along the way during my illness, I came to the conclusion that God was teaching me something and through this experience he was drawing me closer to him. I believe that life's experiences, challenges and struggles make us the person we are destined to be. I know I would not be the person I am today if I had never gone through what I did. As cliché as it may sound, I believe my disease was a wake-up call telling me each day is a gift from God.

When we are not very spiritually aware, we struggle to find meaning and acceptance when first faced with the suffering and pain of a life-altering chronic ailment. There are those who will ask, "Why is this happening to me? What will happen if I die? Is there a God?" or "What have I done to deserve this?"

Doctors usually don't know how to deal with such questions. This is the moment you find yourself turning to spirituality for answers. At first, you discover that it doesn't have the answers for you. It's only later that you find your questions were wrong to begin with. There is no pastor, priest or 'guru' who has answers to those questions, because they are simply not the right questions to ask when you're seeking meaning.

In his book titled *Man's Search for Meaning*, Viktor E. Frankl, a renowned psychiatrist said, "When we are no longer able to change a situation, we are challenged to change ourselves."

In the same book, he also says that, ultimately, we should not ask what the meaning of life is, but instead recognize that it is we who are asked the question. "In a word, each man is questioned by life, and can only answer to life by answering for his own life; to life he can only respond by being responsible."

Frankl believed that love goes very far beyond the physical person of the beloved. It finds its deepest meaning in its spiritual being, his inner self. But his most significant of observations was, "Man is not destroyed by suffering; he is destroyed by suffering without meaning."

Unfortunately, no one tells us these things right in the beginning. Our health care system for the most part discounts the role of spirituality. I think over the centuries, we've come to view science as something that is completely separate from spirituality and to a great extent defined by this separation. Medical technology advances have shifted the focus of medicine from a caring, service-oriented system to a high-tech, cure-oriented model.

When you are a patient with a chronic disease, you are already in a vulnerable position, full of fear and uncertainty of the future and often unable to accept the news. At such a moment, you need to have a more holistic approach to healing.

I suffered from Ulcerative Colitis for many years before I understood this and started to seek the answers and strengthen myself literally from the inside out. In the last ten years I've explored many alternative-healing methods, some that helped and some that didn't, but none helped me as much as exploring my own spirituality.

As I said earlier, one day during one of my worst hospital stays, I found a Pastor praying for me by my bedside. I'm not sure who called for him, or how he came to be there. But sensing him pray for me gave me a glimpse of a source of energy that I could seek and rely on. I began to dig deeper, realizing that there was no quick fix to be found in spirituality. Being closer to and more aware of nature and taking walks helped a great deal. When you are in beautiful natural surroundings, it is hard to ignore the presence of God.

Spirituality and God mean different things to different people, and neither have anything to do with religion. I think religion has political implications, whereas spirituality and God need none. For me, seeking a closer bond with God meant looking at the thoughts in my mind, my self-image, my ego and the emotional patterns I tended to follow and repeat.

From this search, I realized the deep connection between the body, mind and spirit. Years of suppression, then abuse and stress, and then a disconnection between my spirit and body had manifested itself as Ulcerative Colitis in my colon.

If you identify the cause of the problem, you can then start work on determining a path of solution.

I realized I was seeking love from outside of myself. I had been living according to others' expectations of me. All the good energies and positive aspects of me had been buried under an unsteady pile of external negativity and anxiety. I was going through life without actually being completely aware of myself.

I found that this was partly because I had a lot of pent-up fears. They were preventing me from truly experiencing life and being aware. A lot of my energies were tied up in fears: fear of failure, fear of disappointing my husband and my mother, fear of embarrassment, fear of success. If you have to rid yourself of negative energies and free up your good energy to help you heal, you have to let go of those fears you cling to like a security blanket. Fear holds us back from exploring who we truly are and knowing our true purpose. It prevents us from growing, changing our behavior patterns and ourselves. I admit it is one of the hardest things to do, letting go of one's fears, but I also know very well that it is a process integral to living a stronger, happier and honest life. And when you draw upon your faith, fear disappears.

I first began to identify my fears, and then study where they came from. In many ways the process is similar to finding your sources of stress, however, the difference is that your fears are internal, while your stress points are external.

In the early stages of this exploration, I recognized that this was also key to managing stress and getting a grip on remission. I began by watching the thoughts and how I would react to different situations throughout the day. Why did I do and feel in a certain manner, when was it and where was I, who was around me?

I tried to self-reflect, to recognize what the reason was behind a certain emotion or reaction in the situations. I asked myself what were the contributing motivations.

Did I want to make myself feel better? Was it an act of self-preservation? I did this particularly when I felt anxious, annoyed, frustrated or afraid. Over the next few years, I followed a diligent practice of self-reflection and I came to understand myself and what worked or didn't work for me mentally, physically and emotionally.

I began to feel the energy within my body and how I was directing it. I also began to study my emotions rather than simply react to situations. I began to clearly see the root of my UC (stress, inefficient ways of dealing with stress and, worse still, my own faulty thought and behavior patterns). I think yoga helped to some extent because at the start and end of each session, you get a chance to de-clutter your mind of all the extraneous thoughts that have filled it during the day. And the more I practiced de-cluttering, the more I became comfortable with who I am, and the calmer and more aware I became.

I was able to start correcting my responses to situations and my approach to fear and stress, and reducing the number of sources of stress. I knew I was on the right path when I saw how well I did emotionally and physically. My symptoms reduced and, combined with other holistic practices like an organic diet and balancing my body's pH, I found I had discovered how to lead a healthier, happier and more connected life.

One of the greatest insights I've been able to glean from my experience is that the process of maintaining good health and healing ill health extends far beyond removing a disease from the body or simply suppressing its symptoms. It's partly the reason that I have also stayed away from surgery, despite my doctors telling me at one point that I would find it hard to survive without it. When I think about it, I feel if I don't resolve all the external and internal issues that are creating this disease in me, how will removing an organ help? Ill health will simply return in some other form. This is an understanding I've been able to gain only by exploring beyond my physical disease, expanding my consciousness and letting God inspire me to bring more love and compassion to my everyday life. I've improved just by using these enabling tools as opposed to disabling methods in my life with UC.

Disease affects all layers of our being. While I focused on resolving sources of stress and modifying my behavior when I was stressed, I also listened to my body. That is how I arrived at the conclusion that what I ate made a big difference to how well or badly I did. I was able to further narrow down to organic food – and this is what really made a big difference. Being connected to my body allowed me to detect the imbalances in my system. I learned that holistic practices in other cultures have extensively studied these imbalances, what causes them and what resolves them. In Eastern cultures, it's believed that anger and grief are held in cells in particular areas of the body, like the digestive system. These unaddressed emotions cause energy blockages and over time can cause disease.

Cure is not possible for UC, but I firmly believe that there is room for a holistic, spiritually-guided healing. Part of the healing process is to accept the illness and have peace with your life. When we are spiritual, we also use our belief to cope with illness, pain and life's stresses. I believe this is at its very core far more dependable and long-term than any drug or surgery. I don't think I'm alone in this discovery.

There are many studies that support this. A study conducted by Dr. J. W. Yates and others on religion among advanced cancer patients found that those who were spiritual tended to have a more positive outlook, better quality of life and less pain.

Spirituality is an essential part of our life that brings us a sense of stability or "being anchored." It helps us measure our life in terms of a meaningful personal existence, fulfillment of life goals and a feeling that life to that point had been worthwhile, correlated with a good quality of life for patients suffering serious illnesses.

In his report titled "Existential suffering and the

determinants of healing," Eric M. Flanders, a professor of Palliative Medicine at McGill University in Montreal, Canada, says, "Our patients come to us complaining, not of disease, but of their subjective experience of illness. Their quality of life is modified by all domains of personhood – physical, psychological and existential or spiritual."

Professor Flanders goes on to say, "The extremes of human deprivation and the crucible of illness teach us that even in the direst circumstances, peace is possible. What are the variables that influence healing? What is our role as care providers? What is the relevance of these issues to our personal sense of well-being?"

Professor Flander's report explores the concept that quality of life and a sense of being healthy don't necessarily depend on physical well-being. "One may suffer terribly in the absence of physical symptoms; conversely, severe physical decline and pain may be present without anguish or suffering."

There are many other studies as well that have looked at the role of spirituality in managing pain. Many of these have been conducted in patients suffering different forms of cancer, HIV and who have undergone transplant surgeries. And while these don't directly refer to patients of

Ulcerative Colitis, they strongly show the link between spirituality and health. They indicate that spiritual well-being is also related to the ability to enjoy life even in the midst of symptoms, including pain. This suggests that spirituality may be an important clinical target. Results of a pain questionnaire distributed by the American Pain Society to hospitalized patients showed that personal prayer was the most commonly used nondrug method of controlling pain: 76% of the patients relied on it. During this study, 66% of the participants used prayer as a method of pain management more frequently than intravenous pain medication, 62% used it instead of pain injections. Personally, I find that pain medication is very important and should be used, but it is worthwhile to consider other ways to deal with pain as well.

No one can ever be prepared for the tremendous impact, disruption and despair that are brought about by a chronic medical condition. For some people, it creates an inner struggle around beliefs and faith. You may feel abandoned, angry and confused as you try to search for answers to the "why" questions. For others, turning to spiritual practice, meditation or prayer can offer solace and considerable comfort during times when nothing else makes sense. I came to believe that there is a larger purpose and meaning behind the illness and looked for ways to still find gratitude for my life.

CHAPTER 6

MAINTAINING REMISSION

Today, I don't have to take medication when I am in remission. This is unusual because Ulcerative Colitis patients are most often actually prescribed medication particularly for maintaining remission. The only reason I'm able to do fine without medication is because I've been able to find exactly what works for my body and what doesn't. And this is with respect to food, lifestyle, stress and many other aspects that I cover in this book.

There was a time when I had to take more than 35 pills a day. But eventually, I've been able to understand how to maintain my remission without medication. Many of the changes weren't easy, but weaving them into my life and into my normal routine helped greatly in adjusting to them. I view them as I would view taking a shower, brushing my teeth or having breakfast. I slowly removed the tags of "difficult," "selfpity" and other negative associations that we often tend to make. I realized that is the only way to manage the big and small changes that a chronic illness like UC brings to your life. This attitude greatly helps during remission. It helps you to achieve a normal routine with healthy habits and better quality of engagement with the world around you.

Oddly enough, there is no standard definition of remission when it comes to Ulcerative Colitis. There's no medical, endoscopic or histopathological scoring system in UC that marks remission clearly. Definitions vary depending on whether you are talking about remission in the context of treatment trials, the clinical point of view or from a patient's perspective. The reason I will spend some time discussing the lack of a clear definition in this chapter is because I believe it greatly impacts a patient psychologically and it keeps the disease medically ambiguous. The latter in turn makes it difficult for a patient to know what to expect when in remission.

For example, a doctor may choose a particular treatment strategy to achieve remission, which is rarely objective and is usually based on the best balance that they can achieve between symptom control and adverse events from treatment. However, from a patient's perspective, remission usually means being able to lead a certain quality of life. In fact, because of a clear lack of definition for remission there is often a great difference between what a patient has in mind as the goal or expectation from a treatment than that of his doctor.

On another level, researchers working on drug and treatment trials use a definition of remission that would be conducive to drug registration, which is usually the objective of clinical trials.

Therefore, we find there are different definitions of remission. As a patient suffering Ulcerative Colitis, it is important to be aware of each of these in order to set and manage your expectations, understand your doctor's perspective and make informed decisions about treatment choices.

Doctors from leading hospitals and clinics including John Radcliff Hospital, Oxford UK; University of Michigan, Ann Arbor, USA; McGill University Health Centre, Montreal, Canada; Adelaide and Meath Hospital, Trinity College, Dublin, Ireland; et al, wrote extensively about this subject in a paper called "Defining Remission in Ulcerative Colitis" in the Journal of Alimentary Pharmacology and Therapeutics.

According to them, these are the different definitions used for remission in Ulcerative Colitis:

Clinical remission: Used by medical professionals, and meaning cessation of rectal bleeding and normal bowel movement frequency.

Complete remission: Also used in clinical trials to demonstrate safety and efficacy; normal bowel movement frequency and no rectal bleeding as well as a normal or quiescent appearance of the mucosa in a sigmoidoscopy.

Registration remission: Used in trials to gain drug licensure and currently used by regulatory authorities, it requires cessation of rectal bleeding and a sigmoidoscopy score of 0 or 1 of the Mayo Clinic score or Ulcerative Colitis Disease Activity Index.

These definitions do not include the patient's perspective, which may simply mean the ability to enjoy a normal social life, a rewarding career, being able to fulfill parental responsibilities, enjoy family activities without the constant worry of embarrassing moments, pain and other situations associated with UC symptoms.

In the same paper, the authors opine, "It is possible that the absence of a standard definition of remission has contributed to a self-perpetuating cycle of suboptimal therapy in UC." They go on to say that long-term studies show low rates of remission, automatically calling for newer and better treatments, which is something that fuels research from a financial perspective instead of giving it a medical objective.

A clear and widely accepted definition of remission would help a doctor and a patient measure the disease better and choose a course of treatment more accurately. If the definition of remission is clear, it will ensure that the treatment is aligned to that target, and the patient is well aware of what to expect.

A patient's expectations of treatment and remission often differ greatly from those of the doctor. As patients, we sometimes are unable to communicate all our symptoms. In these situations, a doctor unaware of all symptoms may presume that if the patient doesn't talk about it, he or she may not be troubled by it. This may also be because as patients, our attention may be on a certain set of symptoms while we may ignore others because they don't impact us in the context of our daily life. A doctor views your UC mostly from a clinical perspective. Usually, their objective is to implement a treatment that brings endoscopic improvement. Most treatments in UC focus on reducing inflammation of the lining and reducing the severity of ulcers on your colon walls, with as little medicinal side-effects as possible. Whereas, as a patient, our first concerns are:

"Will I be able to get a full night's sleep?" Or "Will I be able to go to my child's school performance?" Or "Can something be done about the horrific stomach cramps?" and other such 'everyday' matters.

It's only when the acute symptoms are taken care of do we start to focus on the long-term, so that we can enjoy longer remissions and avoid flare-ups for as long as possible.

The paper on defining remission points out the difference in perspectives between the medical fraternity and patients' in another very important way. "Many indices contain items which patients do not recognize as being troublesome. Mucus in stools, weight loss and anxiety were among 14 novel items mentioned by patients, but overlooked in indices, while tachycardia, eye symptoms and skin manifestations were incorporated, but of little concern to most patients."

Another startling result pointed out in the article is the difference in the number of flare-ups that an average UC patient in the United States reports and what the number is according to gastroenterologists. A study showed that patients reported, on average, eight (self-defined) flares per year. This was three times the number recognized by physicians. The same study indicates that only 42% of patients believed that being in remission could mean living without symptoms.

When I read this, I'm taken aback. It means gastroenterologists view remission as a period of "no symptoms." Clearly, they underestimate the impact of the disease on our lives and ability to lead a "normal" life.

It brings me to the conclusion that the definition of remission is one that has to be in the context of both the patient and the doctor's treatment objectives. And this should have standardized markers. I know UC affects each person differently and symptoms can vary in severity as well as the fact that not all patients suffer all the symptoms. But there can still be remission markers that are broad and standard.

For me personally, the definition of remission should include a manageable threshold of rectal bleeding and bowel movement frequency. An end to or a reduced sense of the "urgency" that most UC patients suffer from should mark remission. I also believe that doctors should clearly tell us what they mean when they use term like "mild" and "intense."

The following is a definition that my own doctor uses and therefore has greatly contributed to what I define as remission as well: when I have properly formed bowel movements, no urgency and no blood in the stools.

Although I'm often told that this doesn't necessarily mean that the lining of the colon has become perfectly normal, but that it does generally correlate to a healthier state of the colon. Sometimes, doctors may even find some inflammation during remission. This is often taken as a sign that the patient is at a greater risk of colon cancer than another patient who has no inflammation during remission.

Across the board, a gastroenterologist's first goal is to reduce the severity or completely resolve the symptoms of UC and induce remission. By doing so, they believe the body has a chance for the colon to heal. Although most doctors will tell you that a majority of UC patients ultimately undergo surgery to remove the colon, but the first objective in treating UC is to retain the colon. Hence all efforts are focused on relieving it of inflammation and ulcers. Another aim of doctors is to reduce the risk of complications in the long-term, like colon cancer.

Remission and adherence

As with all chronic ailments, the key to maintaining remission lies both in modifying your lifestyle and in following your medication diligently. It's a common human folly: you feel better, you don't sense the symptoms anymore, so you stop following the treatment or skip certain elements of it. Studies support this by finding patients are often at greater risk of a relapse because the success of short-term treatment leads to long-term failure when in the absence of symptoms, patients don't follow their treatment conscientiously.

Apart from classic human behavior, there are many other reasons for lack of adherence to treatment. These include regimen complexity, new patient status, work pressures and shorter disease duration. The studies also showed that men are more likely to skip treatment than women.

Steps I took

As my awareness of the condition grew, I came to peace with the fact that this chronic illness will change my life. For me to expect it not to is being unrealistic and makes it more difficult to adjust to it. In the initial years, the severity of the illness allowed little room for any life outside the hospital. My life was restricted entirely to the home or to the hospital. I spent more time being ill than being in remission during these years. The illness left my body and my mind too weak to understand what was causing my symptoms' severity, or how I should change my lifestyle to support the treatment. I was only taking one day at a time. It was only gradually that I began to stabilize, recognize the role of stress and start to address the issues that were exacerbating my UC.

Over the years, little by little, partially through trial and error and partially by exploring alternative therapies, I learned that I had to change my lifestyle and my eating habits. For example, as I started to get a little better, I brought some stability and independence to my life. I changed my eating habits by listening to my body. I found if I ate smaller quantities instead of three large meals, my stomach did better.

Remission not only gives your colon a chance to heal and be healthier, but it also gives you a chance to understand all the small changes you need to make in your life in order to manage your Ulcerative Colitis more efficiently and effectively. The discipline and habits you establish during remission are the same that will help you stay in remission longer as well.

Each person's needs are different, as are their symptoms and severity. Still, I've listed below the broad methods that I have used to keep myself in remission on a more sustainable basis. These are not foolproof in any way, and while some may work for you, others may not. In still other cases, only a certain combination of these may work.

Medications: These play a very large role in keeping your symptoms under check and bringing your colon relief and if your doctor has put you on a regimen and you have decided to follow it, don't deviate from it or skip a dose. Don't self-medicate. Work with your doctor to determine the best combination of medications for your symptoms, and determine the need for maintenance therapy.

Diet: Doctors will tell you that there is no connection between diet and Ulcerative Colitis. But there is rarely a patient of UC that will tell you they haven't found a direct impact of certain foods on their condition. What is true is that there are no foods that are universally bad for UC patients. While one food may cause no trouble to a UC patient, the same food may severely impact another patient. For example, I have no trouble with dairy products, whereas dairy is a common source of distress to many UC patients. A common-sense solution therefore is to closely monitor your diet. Keep a diary of what you eat throughout the day, so you can eliminate the things that cause you discomfort or a flare-up and focus on things that are easy for you to digest. Some find eating a low-fiber diet is easier on their colon.

It is as important to find out what works for you, as it is to find out what doesn't. Some say that caffeine or artificial sweeteners trigger their flare-ups. Some will tell you beans or popcorn spell trouble; I can tell you they are some of my worst enemies, as is spicy food. Consider limiting foods that produce a lot of gas, which traditionally are beans, legumes and cabbage, but investigate what causes gas for you. Experiment with problem food groups and identify the groups that turn out beneficial. Recent research has found that a diet rich in probiotics and proteins play a very important role in maintaining good health and remission for a UC patient. I'll be covering diet in-depth in a later chapter.

Drink lots of filtered water: Because you're going to the toilet so much, it is important to drink lots of water. It will prevent not only dehydration but also weakness. I like to stress on it being filtered because I've found that it makes a huge difference to me when I have filtered water as opposed to unfiltered water. In many parts of the world, including the United States, unfiltered tap water can contain toxins like fluoride, large amounts of chlorine and heavy metals. We can't always tell how good the water is in our homes, so I always suggest installing a good water filter.

Nutritional supplements: As I said in an earlier chapter, malnutrition is one of the most common problems that accompany Ulcerative Colitis. Ill health, mal-absorption and heavy medication often lead to vitamin deficiencies and weaknesses. Taking multivitamins and other nutritional supplements is therefore essential. Remission is the perfect time to arm yourself because when your colon is not inflamed, it can pursue its normal function of absorbing nutrients from foods. Make sure you select a plant-based multivitamin, not just any, as some multivitamins contain too many preservatives that may cause your colon problems.

Some studies have suggested that omega-3 fatty acids can also reduce Ulcerative Colitis symptoms, along with taking a folic acid supplement. Some studies also show that folic acid supplements may reduce the risk of colon cancer in people with UC. Vitamin D3 and calcium may help prevent bone loss, especially in patients who have been on steroids for long spells. My daily regimen, for example, includes L Glutamine taken daily, Fish Oil, Vitamin D3, protein shakes and maintaining my pH balance and has helped dramatically. I think we often underestimate the power of nutritional supplements.

Surgery: Doctors suggest surgery to patients who don't respond to medication or other treatments. After the entire colon and rectum are removed in a procedure called a total proctocolectomy, another procedure is performed to either reroute bowel movements through a small opening in the abdomen (ileostomy) or to create a pouch using small intestines in an attempt to allow for more normal bowel movements. Since Ulcerative Colitis only occurs in the colon and rectum, this surgery does eliminate the disease, but there can be other issues to deal with afterwards.

Keep a check on stress: Reducing stress and getting emotional support are important aspects of maintaining your remission, not only to prevent flares, but also to maintain overall health. Regular exercise, biofeedback, yoga, tai chi, progressive muscle relaxation, breathing exercises, traveling and socializing can help in a bringing stability and happiness.

The importance of exercise:

I have always loved exercising, so you could say I belong to that group that likes hiking, trekking, walking and working out. But I must tell you, no matter how much you love exercising, when you suddenly drop one-third of your weight and lie for weeks in hospital, barely able carry your own weight to the toilet, exercising is very far from your mind. Nursing yourself slowly back to health during remission is very important. Flare-ups leave us physically and mentally devastated. It is during remission that we get a chance to resume normalcy, and get our bearings back. Whether you have always followed a physical exercise routine or not, always start slowly. You can gradually turn up the intensity as you increase your stamina and strength. And always remember to talk to your doctor before getting started.

Certain exercises tend to be harder on the gastrointestinal tract. Activities with smoother motions, like skating, swimming or cycling tend to be easier on the GI tract than high-impact activities, like running or aerobics. It's also important to choose an activity that you enjoy, so it doesn't become tedious and you are more likely to follow the routine. Personally, I've found yoga to be extremely helpful. It not only helps in keeping my body in better shape, but also helps in de-stressing, refreshing my mind and channeling my positive energy. I find myself always eagerly looking forward to a class.

Another thing that helps me to stick to my physical routine is that I keep myself prepared for all situations – whether I'm going for a walk or going to a yoga class. Keep these points in mind so you eliminate your fear or embarrassment during a flare-up.

Stay close to a toilet: The same principles I mentioned earlier apply to when you plan your workout. At the gym or class, choose a spot near the restroom or a spot near the door so you can get to a toilet fast, when needed.

Warm up and cool down: Remember to spend five to ten minutes at the beginning and end of each workout warming up and cooling down. This gives your muscles and nervous system time to gradually adjust to the change in your activity levels.

Drink lots of filtered water: I can't stress this enough. In any case, it is important for a UC patient to drink lots of water. When you are exercising, it is absolutely imperative. Remember dehydration can worsen UC symptoms. Drink about 16 ounces of water before you start and drink more at the end of a session, even if you aren't feeling thirsty.

Don't overdo it: Overexerting yourself can lead to overheating or dehydration, which can exacerbate Ulcerative Colitis symptoms. Take a break when you feel tired and give yourself time to build up to longer workouts.

Rest when you don't feel well: During Ulcerative Colitis flare-ups, your body is working hard to fight the symptoms of the disease. Don't put more pressure on it. If you have just gone into remission, wait for a few days before resuming your exercise routine.

The secret to successfully maintaining remission is to find the balance between "normal life" and preventive care. Add medication, exercising, diet and other changes into your regular lifestyle so they are indistinguishable from other routine elements of your life. Believe that you can control your symptoms and make your remission last longer.

CHAPTER 7

CROSSING THE ROADBLOCKS

I had been a patient of Ulcerative Colitis for three years when I first started experiencing a strange ache on the left side of my head. My UC was still not under control and I often had to spend several days at a time in the hospital for treatment for severe flare-ups. I was extremely low on energy and still trying to cope with unpleasantness at home. These were indeed dark times. I felt I had no recourse, no refuge and no relief. I was either in the hospital heavily medicated and feeling physically drained or emotionally drained at home.

I didn't pay much attention to the headaches at first. They were just one more pain I tolerated. Then something happened that I couldn't ignore: the vision in my left eye started to get blurry. After a scan, I was told they had found a blood clot in my brain. It was in an area that couldn't be operated on and my only hope would be to take blood thinners, which would hopefully dissolve the clot over time. And while we waited for the blood thinners to work, I ran the risk of the clot affecting the areas of the brain that govern speech and memory; worse still, if the clot were to burst, it would mean sudden death.

At the time I was told, I didn't have the energy or the will to respond. Inside I felt lifeless and in shock. All the physical and emotional turmoil of the previous three years had left me somewhat numb. I used to go through life one day at a time. I had stopped expecting anything from others and I had lowered my expectations of myself. The only thing I could do was manage to live through the day. When I heard the news of the clot, I thought even that was now slipping out of my area of control.

Ironically, I used to be really afraid of injections and needles. But three years of being in and out of hospitals and having it done almost daily had left me partly tough to withstand it and partly desensitized. I wasn't afraid of needles anymore; instead I was ambivalent. I think at first the shock of the blood clot evoked a similar response. As the days went by and I began taking the blood thinners, I started to allow this new complication to actually sink in. Sometimes it helps to cope with bad news if you know why it happened. I asked the doctors what could have caused the blood clot, but they had no answer to offer. Much later, one doctor speculated that there was a chance that the blood clot formed because my hemoglobin levels had been very low and my platelet count had been extremely high for long periods of time. But at the time of diagnosis, nothing was known with certainty: not the cause, nor the risks, nor how long it would take for the course of treatment to take effect, nor if the treatment would work at all or if the blood clot would burst before it could. The only thing certain was that the area was inoperable and the only course of action was to put me on blood thinners and hope for the best. Hopefully the medication would act in time to prevent the clot from bursting, which would cause my brain to bleed and lead to my death.

Ironically, the blood thinners that were administered were given twice a day via injections in my abdomen. Although by this time I had become comfortable with my fear of needles, the injections still hurt quite a bit and each time, the medication caused a burning sensation for almost ten minutes afterwards. Before the discovery of the clot, I thought I had already faced the worst pain and anxiety that fate had in store for me. I didn't think it could get any worse. But it always can, and perhaps that is the rudeness of life; it seems it is also what constantly helps us to push through.

It took one year and three months to dissolve the clot. I lived every day knowing that it could burst any moment and end my life, or worse still leave me speech or memory impaired, or with some other disability. I had to get a brain scan done every three to four months. I remember calming myself and steering myself towards acceptance of whatever God had in store for me instead of wallowing in self-pity.

It feels more comfortable and safer to stay down when you're faced with a roadblock. Sometimes you're just too exhausted physically and mentally to bring yourself to think of how to push through the roadblock. I read somewhere once, "It is much easier to go down a hill than rather up, but always remember that the best view is from the top."

Before I actually got a grasp on how to successfully manage my Ulcerative Colitis condition, I had many dark days, roadblocks and setbacks. In addition to being often bedridden and weak, my life was confined to only the home or the hospital. I still faced physical and psychological abuse in my marriage; I had to go through twelve blood transfusions, the first of which I personally had a tough time accepting. I had started to suffer from the long-term side effects of my UC medication. I was young yet I was barely breathing. I had dreams that I had no place in the future. And still, eventually, these intensely dark days drove me towards the light. They made me thankful for the small things, they taught me to focus on what I had, to not take life's many gifts for granted.

For example, when I finally heard that the clot had dissolved completely, I simply felt humbled and blessed. Words cannot describe how fortunate I felt and thankful I was for God. I am a Christian, but I had never actively practiced my religion or consciously believed in God. In the course of fighting to survive Ulcerative Colitis, I found myself starting to believe in Jesus. Not to beg him for mercy from the pain and suffering, but to draw from him the strength to endure and face the different crisis in my life.

I believe that when you think nothing is going your way, it makes you look at what you still have. The future takes you down a road where you have no control and you can either fight it or let it be.

I think my belief in God during these dark hours rose from seeking the reason for all the pain and suffering. As I said earlier, knowing the reason behind it helps us cope with a situation better. I needed to know why I had undergone these trials. The more I searched and researched, the more I learned. It's not easy to convey in words without sounding cliché or corny, but I had a vision that everything happening in my life was happening for a good reason. And I came to believe that God meant for me to be more appreciative; that I was meant to learn from all this and grow. I had to become a better person for myself and for others.

I saw that my faith and direction began to help me. As the years have gone by, more setbacks, roadblocks and challenges have come. I entered another relationship that at first seemed beautiful but eventually turned ugly.

It took years of listening to my body, research and trial and error methods to find which foods worked best for my body. And during those trials, my body, of course, responded angrily at some times and with relief at other times.

For example, when I started working again, it was difficult yet at the same time it felt like such an accomplishment. It was difficult because it was perhaps the first time I had tried to establish a proper work routine since my diagnosis. Initially, I worked only a few hours a day, only a couple of days a week.

Slowly, I began to push myself a little. That's what impediments do. They come without warning but as you surmount each one, it gives you the confidence that perhaps you could surmount another. Even today, there are times when I have a bad tummy day. In the early years, it would leave me devastated and confined to my home. But now, I find that if I can just get myself to work or to the friend I'm supposed to meet, my stomach will stabilize itself in an hour or so.

It felt good to be able to work again; not just because of the Ulcerative Colitis but because I was finally able to be guilt-free. It was the ability to surmount the impediments that gave me the confidence to pursue my dreams and the hope of being a productive part of society again.

While I may sound like one, but I'm not a shiny happy evangelist. I know very well the bad hand that I was dealt, but I'm thankful for it - it has made me a realist as well as an optimist in equal measures. I was never the sort who would see a silver lining in each cloud or say that the glass was always half-full. I call myself a realist and an optimist now because even today, the realist in me looks at that glass being half-empty, while the optimist says, well, now I have a chance to fill it up with whatever I choose.

In the ten years that I have lived with UC, I have fought intensely to regain control of my life, find purpose, meaning and reconstruct myself as a more aware and complete human being. I once read somewhere, "You are what you eat." I think the same is startlingly true when it comes to our relationships, environment and attitude. You are what you believe. This isn't to say that I am preaching some flaky concept about "mind over matter," or the idea that you can just "think" your illness away. Back in the days when I was taking anywhere between 15 to 30 pills a day and being administered intravenous steroids, I would have found it hard to believe that there would come a day when I would be able to manage my chronic disease well enough to not have to be on meds 24-7. I didn't get here because of a divine miracle, or simply by hypnotizing myself into believing I didn't have UC - I did it by looking in the mirror, having faith in God's design and drawing strength from it to accept the fact that the glass was half empty because I was meant to fill it with something wonderful and empty it of ills.

Acceptance, you will often hear, is one of the biggest transitions anyone can make. For example, with a limited amount of energy, the sudden onslaught of cramps, numerous toilet calls in a day and never quite knowing when any or all of these symptoms would hit meant that my plans could change from one moment to another with little or no warning. But it also meant I had to learn to be more flexible with my expectations of myself and my plans for the day. I trained myself to not get deeply disappointed or feel crushed when plans changed or got cancelled.

On many occasions, when I was very weak, I would accept that with reduced energy I could only do a certain amount that day, sometimes nothing at all. I began to prioritize what was important to me and not to dwell too much on what was not important. Realizing these simple things prevents me from getting stressed, which is one of my top causes of a flare-up.

Each setback during these ten years, as painful and exhausting as they were, eventually helped me hone the skill of finding my center amidst the metaphorical storm. It helped me identify the things I didn't want to be part of my personality or life and the things I wanted to incorporate.

In the initial years, I remember spending a lot of time being really jealous of healthy people. I was young and completely debilitated by my UC. While others enjoyed going out, eating and drinking whatever they wanted, I was either confined to the bed and toilet or I had to extensively think over a plan a hundred times just go out for a lunch. I remember thinking what do people who say "I'm dying" when they only have a bad cold know what it's like to actually feel when you're truly near death. As people with horrible chronic ailments, we tend to live in a bubble and think of ourselves only in terms of our sickness.

But gradually, I've come to realize that we aren't in competition. What kind of community would we be if all we did was sit around and try to one-up each other about who felt the worst? Pain is pain. It comes to everyone in varying forms. Some have physical pains, others have emotional or psychological ones. Being closer to God has also helped me recognize that no life goes un-signed by pain. And for the person who is suffering it, it is no less important than anyone else's.

There are some other ways in which I cope with setbacks and impediments. These are things I've learned from experiences in other aspects of my life – from work, relationships, friendships and family. But they are just as applicable to understanding how to deal emotionally and psychologically with the setbacks you undergo as a UC patient.

In 1985, in a paper titled "Putting a Premium on Regret," economist and former vice president of the Ford Foundation, David E. Bell, introduced the "Disappointment Theory." According to this, we experience disappointment when a situation that has an uncertain outcome ends up producing a result that is worse than we had expected. He further suggested that we're most likely to be disappointed when we are seeking a positive outcome, when we feel that we deserve this positive outcome, when the failure to achieve that outcome is a surprise and when the failure is outside of our personal control. When I first read this, I thought, *My God! He's writing what we as UC patients feel so often!* I think sometimes we get so wrapped up in a disease that we forget there are principles and strategies that apply to other situations that could be just as effective for a patient suffering a chronic ailment like UC.

The fact is that the impact of disappointment reaches beyond just feeling sad. It impairs our decision-making abilities. For example, an article on the subject in the magazine *Psychology Today* states that economists find that people who are experiencing the emotion of disappointment are more likely to be prone to the so called "endowment effect." It goes on to explain: "According to the endowment effect, people are more likely to want to demand more money to sell an item they already have than they are to spend in order to acquire the very same item." The more we think about giving up an item we already own, the more our minds see its value. However, when people are in a sad mood, they are less likely to show the endowment effect.

In a 2011 experiment conducted by Luis Martinez, Marcel Zeelenberg and John Rijsman, participants assigned values to how much they were willing to accept selling a mug they already were told they owned compared to how much they were willing to pay to buy the same mug. During the study, the participants were first asked to write about recent experiences they had had that could be categorized under regret or disappointment. The objective of this exercise was to evoke those emotions in each participant before they were asked to make decisions on the value of items.

The study observed that people project their own negative emotions onto the objects they possess. It theorized that as humans, the more we regard an item as a reflection of our identity (e.g., an item with a team's insignia), the more likely it is we'll devalue that item when we're in a bad mood. As it turned out, the participants in the study conducted by Martinez and his collaborators assigned lower values to items they had in their possession when experiencing the emotion of disappointment.

In order to prevent disappointments and setbacks from getting the better of us, experts suggest the following strategies. Some of these I arrived at during my own journey, other's I came to know of from experts in the fields of psychology and management.

Try a bit of "retroactive pessimism:" Psychologists suggest that if you tell yourself that you didn't really expect to win, as time goes by, the new memory will replace the original, more painful memory. This helps in preventing your sense of disappointment from impacting other aspects of your personality like self-esteem, hopefulness and decision-making abilities.

It doesn't mean you are in denial, it just means you are looking at the same event in hindsight from a different perspective.

Increase your tolerance level of setbacks: To prevent setbacks from leading to pessimism, lower your negative reaction to them a little. Try to feel less daunted and less stressed by each hurdle because if you feel more daunted, you're making it harder for yourself to manage the next one.

Don't let disappointment skew your self-worth: Think of it like this: If your favorite sports team lost a championship, you don't go put your much-loved team collectables up on eBay, do you? In the same sense, don't let an impediment or disappointment cloud your judgment of yourself.

Be realistic about what you control: If your expectations in love, work or maintaining your health chronically fail to materialize, make an honest appraisal of what you may need to change in yourself. Learn to differentiate what you can control or change and what you cannot. Be aware of the trade-off you're making when you cannot have control over something or change yourself.

Control your identification with a lost cause: This is particularly true of jobs, relationships, diets and other things we hold on to despite knowing they are doing us no good. There's nothing wrong with giving something another go (whether it be a job, relationship or something else) but if it is impairing your daily happiness, you need to find other ways to fulfill the need.

Use humor: This helps to dissolve the tension that hard situations bring. Instead of wallowing in self-pity, it's better to laugh it off in self-deprecation.

Do something meaningful often: Do something that gives you a sense of accomplishment often. Set goals to help you look toward the future with meaning and to balance out the lows you may feel from time to time.

Get connected: Building strong, positive relationships at work and with loved ones and friends can provide you with needed support and acceptance in both good times and bad.

Maintain hope: You can't change what's happened in the past, but you can always look toward the future. Accepting and even anticipating change makes it easier to adapt and view new challenges with less anxiety.

Write it down: Think back on how you've coped with hardships in the past. You might write about past experiences in a diary to help you identify good and bad behavior patterns.

Embrace creativity regularly: Be it music, cooking or pottery, engaging yourself creatively has a significant effect on your ability to manage impediments or crisis situations.

CHAPTER 8

IMPURITIES OF LOVE: THE IMPACT OF TOXIC RELATIONSHIPS ON HEALTH

Fighting like dogs, cold wars, the silent treatment, stomping off, slamming doors, feeling like you are never reaching a resolution... most of us who have gone through bad relationships know this really well. It feels like you are drowning in a pit of tar: nothing you do seems to help, you don't feel loved or cared for and there comes a point at which you don't have the energy even to think clearly much less to want to do anything different. What we often don't realize is that living in a relationship like this has a negative impact not only on the health of the relationship but also on our own physical health.

It's ironic that as a society we spend so much time being concerned about toxins in our water, food and air, but we are quite blind to the toxins in our relationships. Being exposed to toxic relationships can be just as bad as being exposed to toxins in fast foods or the environment; the impact takes place slowly but very deeply and for over a long period of time. An unhealthy relationship spreads its illness into our bodies, our minds and our emotions.

People think being alone makes you feel lonely. I don't think that's true at all. To the contrary, I believe being surrounded by the wrong people to be the loneliest situation in the world. I know this most intimately. I was at my worst point in Ulcerative Colitis and yet that didn't stop my partner from physically, mentally and sexually abusing me. It was unbearable and yet at the time I just couldn't find the strength to get out of the situation. I remember once how hard my body shook with the familiar mix of fear, disgust and anger. However, the truth is that no matter how familiar the emotion is, the toll it takes on your body and mind gets worse with each incident.

The psychological, emotional and physical impact isn't just a conjecture. Countless studies have substantiated this observation; among these, the most landmark work is the Whitehall II study conducted by Sir Michael Marmot and his team at the University College in London. It began in 1985 and was conducted over a period of twelve years, with more than 10,000 men and women from the British civil services between the ages of 35 and 55. Researchers controlled for psychological factors like depression, anxiety and stress as well as lifestyle, social demographics (age, marital status, sex, employment status) and biological factors like high blood pressure, diabetes, obesity and cholesterol levels. The context of the study was heart disease and its primary objective was to measure how negative close relationships impacted the development and risk of heart disease. During the course of the study, the volunteers were given questionnaires designed to evaluate the negative aspects of their closest personal relationships. Researchers divided responses into those where the closest relationship identified was the spouse/partner versus non-spouse/non-partner. Spouses were the first closest relationship for 64% percent of the responses. The researchers further categorized the responses by the type of relationship the volunteers shared with these spouses. They defined the two types as:

a) One that was confiding, featured emotional support, was a self-esteem builder and where the two shared values and interests.

b) One that gave practical support The researchers found that certain groups of people were more likely than others to experience negative close relationships. These included younger participants, women, men whose jobs were considered lower economic jobs and people who were never married. In addition, researchers also found that relationships that involved people who had earlier been a divorcee or a widow had a higher risk for cardiac events if the relationship was negative.

The trouble with toxic relationships is that they can take many forms: a toxic partner, friend, an unhealthy parent-child relationship or toxic coworkers. But of them all, the largest influence on health is from a toxic partner.

Another study, published in early 2012 in the Proceedings of the National Academy of Sciences and carried out by The School of Medicine at the University of California, Los Angeles, found that stress from sour relationships that aren't terminated can cause inflammation, which in turn leads to a variety of health issues like heart disease, cancer and high blood pressure. The main focus of the study was to measure the increase of proteins responsible for inflammation in the body when the participant is undergoing stress in a relationship. During this study, 122 healthy participants were asked to keep a diary, highlighting any stressful incidents they had with their partners and how they dealt with it. They were also given math quizzes and public-speaking assignments under laboratory conditions. A few days later, the inside of their cheeks were swabbed to check the level of cytokines (the proteins that influence the inflammatory response of the body) and the results showed that those who suffered from the most stress had higher levels of pro-inflammatory cytokines.

Stepping out of the bubble

The first thing we have to do is recognize when we are in a toxic relationship. During my marriage, I didn't truly recognize the amount of stress I was under, nor could I fathom the extent of physical damage it was causing me. It was only later that I caught on to a pattern of UC flare-ups. When I stayed with my partner, I'd have horrible attacks of UC; however, when I'd go away, I would be so much better.

Now I can tell when a relationship is toxic and dysfunctional. Of course, no relationship is blissful and conflict-free all the time, but there are certain indicators that should ring the alarm bells for you. Also, I believe it is important to admit that there are two sides to a relationship, so this is not a blame-game. These questions are merely for oneself to understand what is happening in a relationship and how one reacts and responds - whether that in turn is making things worse. I once read a magazine article by Dr. Matthew Sherrigan, a consultant psychologist, where he suggests asking the following questions:

1) When you're with your partner, do you usually feel content and motivated or do you feel unfulfilled and drained?

2) After spending time with him/her, do you usually feel better or worse about yourself?

3) Do you feel physically or emotionally safe with this person, or do you feel threatened or in danger?

4) Is there a fairly equal give-and-take in the relationship? Or do you feel like you're always giving and he/she is always taking?

5) Is the relationship characterized by feelings of security and contentment or drama and resentment?

6) Do you feel like he/she is happy with who you are? Or do you feel like you have to change to make him/her happy?

I think anyone would agree that a healthy and thriving relationship is characterized by compassion, security, safety, freedom of thinking, sharing, listening, mutual love/caring, healthy debate/disagreements and respectfulness, especially when there are differences of opinion, whereas toxic relationships are characterized by insecurity, abuse of power and control, neediness, demandingness, selfishness, insecurity, self-centeredness, criticism, negativity, dishonesty, distrust, demeaning comments/attitudes or jealousy.

This is exactly how I've come to observe the influence my relationships have had on my life. The healthy ones have always left me happy and energized while the toxic ones have left me depressed, depleted and sick.

What it does to the body

I've said before that stress triggers the body's "fight or flight" mechanism, signaling it to produce hormones like cortisol and adrenaline. Digestion slows, heart rate speeds up and your muscles are tensed and ready for action. If you truly needed to fight or run for your life, you'd be ready to go. In hindsight, I know that during my marriage, I had fallen into a chronic stress pattern, so my body never really fully relaxed, taking a heavy toll on my organ functions in the process.

Chronic stress has been linked to a variety of health problems, including chronic pain, headaches, stomach aches, sleep problems, depression and weakening of the immune system. It can worsen pre-existing conditions as well, like stomach and bowel problems, psoriasis, acne and asthma. Researchers have also found links to high blood pressure, heart attacks, atherosclerosis and blood clots.

According to a study published in 2000 in the Journal of the American Medical Association, women who reported moderate to severe marital strain were 2.9 times more likely to need heart surgery, suffer heart attacks or die of heart disease than women without marital stress. These findings held true even when researchers adjusted for other factors such as age, smoking habits, diabetes, blood pressure and bad cholesterol levels. Women in cohabitating relationships who were involved with severely stressful affairs also had a higher risk of heart problems.

These results were echoed by another study published in the American Journal of Cardiology in 2006 that showed that the four-year survival rate of those with both severe heart disease and poor marriages was 42%, compared to 78% among patients with both milder heart disease and good marriages.

The impact on the immune system

We know that Ulcerative Colitis is a disease related to an impaired immune system. When I look at this fact and look at the research that has found the disruptive influence of marital conflict on the immune system, I'm not surprised. When I finally filed for a divorce, I had realized deep inside the role that my marriage was playing in keeping me sick.

However, it was only a very deeply felt notion. When I did research while writing this book, I was relieved to find this wasn't simply a notion, but actually substantiated by research and statistics. Today I feel I have a stamp of credibility to what I thought was only a conjecture on my part, no matter how real that conjecture is to me.

According to a 1993 article in the journal *Psychosomatic Medicine*, newlywed couples involved in a 30-minute heated discussion of marital problems tended to have relatively poorer immunological responses, unlike couples engaged in positive or problem-solving behaviors.

Some of the most fascinating research in the connection between physical health and marital stress comes from Ohio State University by Ronald Glaser, an immunologist, and his wife Jan Kiecolt-Glaser, a member of the psychiatry department in the same university. They were particularly interested in the connection between marital stress and immunity. It is already known that when we experience a high level of stress, our body's ability to produce white blood cells (our natural protectors against viruses and cancer) and antibodies significantly drops. They further conducted a series of carefully constructed studies to find that people in marriages that featured a high level of hostility, contempt and fights took two full days longer to heal from wounds than couples who experienced and showed less animosity during their arguments.

All of these studies are great as an affirmation of what I thought as a layperson. But there is a greater significance when I look at it from the perspective of an Ulcerative Colitis patient. It implies that when we are fighting this disease, men and women who carry the extra baggage of a toxic relationship need to not only remove themselves from that environment, but allow themselves more time to recover from flare-ups and possibly look at additional medical and emotional support systems. Simply put, we need to take even greater care than the patient next to us who may come from a healthier personal environment.

Slower disease recovery

There is another very specific fallout of bad relationships: they slow down the body's ability to recover from disease. Over a series of flare-ups, I noticed that when I would return from the hospital and I would be back in the unpleasant and stressful environment of my marriage, healing took longer and became increasingly difficult each time. Stress not only increased the severity of the flare-ups, but it also reduced my body's ability to heal post treatment.

A study published in 2009 in a cancer journal demonstrated how marital distress was associated with worse recovery graphs of breast cancer survivors. Patients who participated in the survey and came from toxic relationships had not only higher levels of stress but eventually showed more impaired functioning than those who came from healthy marriages. There's another interesting observation the researchers made: participants who were in a bad relationship tended to be less compliant with medical regimens or adhering to healthy dietary habits.

Psychological and emotional impacts

Negative behaviors during conflict in relationships, such as resentment and criticism, have an awful impact on our mental and emotional state as well as our physical being. Each time we get a taunt or barb, it chips away at our self-confidence and we invariably react by becoming a shade more vulnerable.

I read an old article in the *Journal of Health and Social Behavior* when doing my research for this book and found an interesting observation: single people tend to have better mental health than those who remain in a tumultuous relationship!

Sometimes, we tend to go from one bad relationship to another, afraid of being lonely and desperately seeking the stability of a good relationship. But in my experience, going through too many breakups is even worse for our mental health than staying single.

The *Journal of Epidemiology and Community Health* published a paper by researchers who studied more than 2,000 men and women over a period of six years who went through several break-ups. They found that women in the study particularly tended to have worse mental health than women in the controlled group who remained single all their lives.

It can be difficult to wipe a person out of your life, especially if the relationship has been long and not constantly toxic. However, you really do owe it to yourself and to your family to try and extract yourself, or at least keep your distance. Toxic relationships just aren't worth the stress (or the health implications) that they could bring.

To stay or go

I think for every individual, the decision to stay or leave a relationship is an extremely difficult one. I remember when trouble initially started between my partner and I, my first strategy was to avoid the things that could possibly cause conflict. When that didn't succeed, I tried to change myself. In a situation of extreme distress, you feel you lack control over the other person. That was how I felt and I thought that the only thing I could change was myself. So I tried that, but that didn't help greatly either. Perhaps what needed to change were the behavior patterns we both had: controlling, demanding and hostile behavior from him, and responding with greater tolerance and self-sacrificing on my part. I wouldn't stand up for myself. It was hard for me to vocalize that I was not okay being physically and mentally abused, and being ill with Ulcerative Colitis just made it harder for me to make any decision.

At such times of extreme stress, if you continue to remain in a toxic environment without resolving it, sooner or later any counter-measures you take to feel better will stop helping. But ultimately, I knew what I had to do.

Even after my divorce, it took some years to truly move on and shake free from having borne the burden of a toxic relationship. Holding grudges only extended the period of mourning of the relationship. My forays into spirituality and my belief in Jesus helped a great deal to resolve the years of grief, and remove its control over my disease. Letting go of it allowed me to start to heal, physically and emotionally.

I realized the solution to a toxic relationship was to not be with the person who was causing me stress, but to change my situation and create a new paradigm for my life, adapt to it and accept Jesus into my life.

Changing how you choose a partner

What I find most puzzling is how perfectly intelligent and accomplished women and men often have the propensity to corner themselves in a relationship where they are constantly criticized and considered inadequate. I believe they internalize this feedback because it comes from someone they love and desperately need approval from.

I watched a film recently called "Perks of Being a Wallflower," where the protagonist says: "We accept the love we think we deserve." While I partly agree, there is a part of me that doesn't find it acceptable. I believe it is a tendency that needs to be corrected. It is only when we break free from the self-created definition of love that is causing us pain that we can lead a healthier life.

Choosing a partner requires greater thought than we often give. In my earlier relationships I was unable to tell my partners what I wanted. They didn't know how to deal with my UC, or perhaps they didn't truly want to. Today, I wouldn't go out with a person who I think isn't psychologically, emotionally and physically able to deal with the uncertainties my illness brings in my life. In my mind, it's finally clear that I've had my life-threatening experiences and I don't need a relationship to bring me another.

For example, on a very shallow level, I know my partner has to be sensitive to my diet requirements, the need to be close to a bathroom, the possibilities of a flare-up altering an evening plan. These are just the basics.

For me, Ulcerative Colitis not only forced me to learn how to listen to my body, but also to re-examine how my mind processed the information and how I arrived at these choices. Being a sensitive person, I believe I might be setting myself up for more grief that could be actually avoided.

As highly sensitive people, we are very gentle and often quiet on the outside but highly expressive, emotional and passionate on the inside. So when we meet someone we like, instead of a spark, it's like a bonfire of attraction and energy. We then have to struggle emotionally and psychologically to get a grasp on this rollercoaster experience. It's easy to confuse chemistry, love and a soul mate. The reality is that a fiery romance is often a sign that the relationship will eventually self-combust. Heightened emotions are characteristically unstable. It is like working in a lab with extremely powerful elements and not knowing really how to use them and in what measure. It also makes us blind to the unhealthy aspects of our partner. And when we do start to recognize these, we're already deep in a toxic relationship.

Highly sensitive people are natural nurturers with a driving desire to foster others' personal growth. I think this is one of the strongest patterns I found when looked back on my relationships. We are the world's counselors, finding great personal fulfillment in helping and encouraging our partner. As highly sensitive individuals, we are well attuned to sensing another person's deeper feelings, which are often painful. So we respond with tremendous compassion; we're so adept at empathizing that we feel others' emotions even more than our own. Normal people I think have a shield around them that protects them from the world's rawness. But like a person turned inside-out, a highly sensitive person wears his or her sensitivity on the outside, showing their soft side to the world and absorbing every nuance. This can make us feel overwhelmed and it can add stress that we don't even recognize, making us put others ahead of ourselves and ignore our own needs. I think, in my relationships, I completely lost touch with my own needs at one point.

I realized somewhere along the way that I had to find the balance between helping others and helping myself, so that I could enjoy the fulfillment of supporting other people while still looking after myself. That meant establishing and expressing clear boundaries with others so that any kind of unhealthy behavior was not tolerated. Even today, this is a process that I have to follow very consciously and it is easy for me to slip back into the mode where I put my own needs last.

However, I remind myself that setting boundaries and expressing my needs clearly detracts unhealthy people from seeking me out. I'm less attracted to them and it allows me to attract people who are healthy enough to be there for me as well, which is most important. I know now that is where a stress-free and deeper sense of love comes from.

Toxic friendships

Unlike when we are children, many of our adult friendships are born of convenience. I think to a great extent this is because they are not so much a product of personal choice as they are a result of circumstances or happening.

For example, I go to a certain yoga class, so I have friends there; or I live close to my friends, so we often meet. But when our personal circumstances change, the conditions of our friendships can also change, leading us to a point where we are forced to reconsider why we were putting our energy into it. A sign of a friendship being born of convenience appears when I ask myself for example, *"If I were to move, how often would my friends meet up with me?"* And the answer is: *not often.*

For me, it was my belief in Jesus that led me to want to live authentically. And one important aspect of living authentically is living in truth. From a friendship standpoint, this means not living in a state of denial about the conditions that surround that friendship. It also means not passively accepting the negative aspects that we would be better off avoiding.

Relationships of convenience or fair-weather friends by definition prompt us to give a lot of leeway to society's faults and people's shortcomings. But constantly doing that unwittingly leads us to compromise ourselves. Taking the time to examine our friendships - sorting out the synergies between our experience with another person and our own values is key to living in a way that is both authentic and evolving.

In the end, I feel we encounter so many different relationships in our lifetimes, all of which change the people we are in one way or another.

As I look back on my life, I find that perhaps I could not always choose who I fell in love with, nor could I change the people I fell in love with when things went wrong. I can, however, be happy with who I am as an individual and stay firm in what I want in life and what I believe to be love.

CHAPTER 9

SURGERY: THE BIG QUESTION

Finally, more than anything, I have come to peace with this entire experience because I know that Jesus is in control. I feel his presence every day in a quiet but reassuring way in every choice I make and every action. There are two stories in the Bible that have particularly moved me and inspired me to take control of my Ulcerative Colitis, rather than let it control me. Most of all they have led me away from a point of severity where surgery was increasingly becoming the only option to a state where I no longer have to take medication on a daily basis.

Later Jesus went to Jerusalem for a special Jewish festival. In Jerusalem, there is a pool with five covered porches. In the Jewish language it is called Bethzatha. This pool is near the Sheep Gate. Many sick people were lying on the porches {beside the pool}. Some of the people were blind, some were crippled, and some were paralyzed. There was a man lying there who had been sick for 38 years. Jesus saw the man lying\ there. Jesus knew that the man had been sick for a very long time. So Jesus asked the man, "Do you want to be well?" The sick man answered, "Sir, there is no person to help me get into the water when the water starts moving. I try to be the first person into the water. But when I try, another person always goes in before I can." Then Jesus said, "Stand up! Pick up your bed and walk." Then immediately the man was well. The man picked up his bed and started walking. The day all this happened was a Sabbath day. So some Jews said to the man that had been healed, "Today is the Sabbath. It is against our law for you to carry your bed on the Sabbath day." But the man answered, "The person (Jesus) that made me well told me, 'Pick up your bed and walk.'" The Jews asked the man, "Who is the person that told you to pick up your bed and walk?" But the man that had been healed did not know who the person was. There were many people in that place, and Jesus had left. Later Jesus found the man at the temple. Jesus said to him, "See, you are well now. But stop sinning or something worse may happen to you!" Then the man left and went back to those Jews. The man told them that Jesus was the one that made him well. John 5: 1-15

Now, I do realize that we don't live in a world of such dramatic miracles anymore and that sometimes, we may need more than faith to heal ourselves, but the message of this passage is so much greater than its literal import.

Jesus asks, "Would you like to get well?" On the face of it, this is such a redundant question. Who wouldn't want to be well? And after all, the man had come to the pool to be healed. But like the saying, "You can lead a horse to water but you can't make it drink," this story also suggests you have to take responsibility of yourself. We, ourselves, are our biggest obstacle in life. If we can overcome our own hesitations, insecurities and disbeliefs in ourselves, we could actually move mountains.

"Do I want to get well?" When you have been sick for many years, for some it becomes easier to remain sick than risk the effort to get better. In a book titled What Jesus Did, the author writes, "You think I might have to change. I might have to give up my excuses. I might have to adapt to a different lifestyle. I might have to give up blaming others for my problems. I might have to take some responsibility for my own condition. Jesus asked the question because, in this case, it was the real disease. As the man shows by the end of the story, he wasn't ready to take responsibility for anything."

Faith has taught me to rely on God, who lives in our hearts and creates a source of power and a set of abilities within us. It has taught me to not feel so helpless and forsaken because He is always with us.

In Matthew, Chapter 17, verses 14-21, when Jesus and the apostles Peter, James and John returned to the crowds, a man came and knelt in front of Jesus. "Lord, do have pity on my son," he said, "for he has seizures and is suffering greatly. He often falls into the fire or into the water. I brought him to your disciples but they could not heal him."

"You really are an unbelieving and perverse generation," Jesus replied. "How long shall I stay with you? How long shall I put up with you? Bring the boy here to me." Jesus rebuked the demon, and it came out of the boy, and he was healed at that moment.

Afterwards, the disciples approached Jesus privately and asked, "Why couldn't we drive it out?"

"Because you have so little faith," replied Jesus. "Truly I tell you, if you have faith as small as a grain of mustard-seed you can say to this mountain, 'Move from here to there,' and it will move. Nothing will be impossible for you."

For me it wasn't simply that I got up one day and chose to be well, so I became well. It has been a gradual, increasingly rewarding journey of high awareness to become well. I took my health into my own hands; I became truly responsible for myself by rooting out the causes of ill health, by adopting new practices that brought my digestive system to a better state of functioning and by believing that I can be in better health without getting my entire colon removed.

For each of us who suffer from Ulcerative Colitis, the decision to have surgery or not is an extremely personal one. According to an article published a few years ago in the *New York Times*, there are 1.4 million Americans with inflammatory bowel disease; about 500,000 of these have Ulcerative Colitis. The same article goes on to say that 20 percent of these Ulcerative Colitis patients will eventually have surgery. Surgery in the case of this disease is not exactly a minor operation. In fact, it is a fairly complex and long procedure that is sometimes split into 3 separate stages because it involves removal of the colon and rectum, creation of a pouch to store waste, construction of a temporary opening (ileostomy) in the abdominal wall, then closure of that opening so the patient can go to the toilet normally. It is an extremely difficult surgery that requires highly-skilled surgeons, and even though it promises freedom from the pains of UC, it is in itself a long and daunting ordeal that brings patients as much fear as it brings hope. There's fear of incontinence with the pouch and very loose motions for the first few weeks and fear of death from the surgery, fear of disfigurement, among many other anxieties. For women, there is possible formation of scar tissue due to surgery which interferes with the reproductive system and the ability to have children.

However, for a majority of patients, surgery is a choice driven not by saving their life but for improving its quality. This elective nature of the surgery makes it very difficult to make the decision.

There are doctors who are pro-surgery because they believe it is better than forever being on medicines with side effects and because some are highly-skilled surgeons trained to believe in resolving the body's issues with surgery. There are other medical professionals who believe there is nothing better than the organs nature has developed in the human body. They will suggest it is better to work towards avoiding surgery and try to keep the symptoms under control with medication with least side effects, prolong remission as much as one can and ease the pressures off the organ than remove the organ itself. These doctors will also tell you that your quality of life in remission is no different to the quality of life you have after surgery.

The surgery itself

There are two types of surgery performed to treat Ulcerative Colitis:

Proctocolectomy and ileostomy: Here, the anus, rectum and colon are removed, a small hole is made on the right side of your stomach wall, just below your belly button. This allows surgeons to place the end of your small intestine at the opening, enabling your body to eliminate wastes into a bag that is worn outside the hole. No one realizes you are wearing a bag as there is no smell and it's well hidden under your clothes.

For some patients of Ulcerative Colitis, surgery is a necessity for survival and is not an option. When the colon's lining becomes cancerous or close to being perforated from ulcers, the operation becomes a life-saving procedure that cannot be avoided or postponed. It is also performed as an emergency measure when there is severe expansion of the colon wall leading to increasing gases and bacteria in the colon. Or, when there is heavy bleeding from the colon and the body is not responding to medication or being able to cope despite blood transfusion.

Restorative Proctocolectomy: Developed over two decades ago, it is a two-step procedure and it doesn't involve removing the anus and the muscles that control the anus. Instead, a pouch known as the J-pouch is created from the small intestines and attached to the anus. This pouch needs time to heal so an external pouch is attached to your abdomen for 10 to 12 weeks. When the J-pouch is healed, the external pouch is removed.

With both procedures, you are medically considered cured of Ulcerative Colitis because the part of the body that caused its symptoms is gone. If you have restorative proctocolectomy, you eliminate the body's waste through the anus normally, though your trips to the toilet may be as often as six times a day. Restorative proctolectomy. has many risks including an obstruction of the bowel, resulting in bowel scars or adhesions that can occur because of surgery - although lately, the use of ultrasound activated scalpels has lowered the risk of complications.

The pouch made from the small intestines may not hold and may develop leaks, leading to another surgery to construct a permanent external pouch. The J-pouch can become inflamed, an issue that has been found to happen in 30% of cases where patients have elected a restorative proctocolectomy.

Long-term results of having a restorative proctocolectomy are still considered uncertain, though more recent studies have shown that many patients have fared well over the long term.

It's important to know that the outcome after surgery may not always be exactly like a person with a normal digestive system. You may still be going to the toilet several times a day, but you won't have the pain, bleeding, inflammation and other symptoms and life-disrupting issues associated with Ulcerative Colitis. Studies also show that a restorative proctocolectomy has increasingly been the choice of surgery for the last 20 years, and it's particularly popular as an elective procedure. There is evidence that fertility is reduced to about 50% in women who undergo this operation. Studies also show that the overall rate of failure of restorative proctocolectomy after ten years of having undergone it, rises to 15%. More than 50% of failures are caused by sepsis, followed by poor function, followed by mucosal inflammation and a small percentage of the failures are due to formation of a malignant tumor.

Still, there are thousands of testimonials in books, blogs, websites and journals from patients who have seen a dramatic and positive change in their lives after surgery. These are usually accompanied by narratives about varied degrees of difficulty and the challenges of adjusting to a pouch and complications that arise from time to time related to the pouch. But, more or less, they all seem to be eventually happy having undergone surgery.

In my case, I decided against the surgery. I know this is an unusual and less common decision, and one that was made despite being told at one point that surgery may be the only option. But I managed to fight back in my own way. I think too often we give up on this fight. We yield to a relatively easier option. I think one of the most important lessons I have gained and that I really want to share is that decisions regarding your health cannot be based just on medical terms. You have to consider emotional and psychological motivations as well.

There are some extremely hard questions you have to ask yourself:

1. Are you willing to take responsibility of your body?

2. Do you want to be healed?

3. Does staying sick serve some ulterior but much-needed purpose?

4. Regardless of whether you decide on surgery or not, are you willing to do whatever it takes to get better?

5. Do you know the emotional and psychological toll any complex surgery takes?

And do you know how you will deal with this?

The most critical decisions in life are extremely personal. But in the case of surgery for Ulcerative Colitis, there is just so much pro-surgery talk in the public domain that it can trick you into thinking that it is the logical and most obvious course of action to take. As you consider my personal situation, you may find that there is perhaps another path to healing.

CHAPTER 10

RIGHT PEOPLE, RIGHT CHOICES

I once read a passage that left a very deep impact on me: "Keep away from people who try to take away and talk you out of your ambitions." Really great people make you feel that you, too, can become great. Surround yourself with dreamers, doers, believers and thinkers – but most of all surround yourself with those who see greatness within you.

There are two kinds of people in this world: those you choose to have in your life and those you don't. There was a time when this was not as clear and simple to me as I now put it to you. I spent a great part of my life wasting vast amounts of energy trying to impress, please and keep people happy who had absolutely no interest in me or my well-being.

We all do this at some point or another out of obligation, politeness or an inability to say 'no' and perhaps because we have latent insecurities that make us want to please and earn approval. In fact, the latter often makes us overcompensate. We go out of our way to belong and be loved. So we find ourselves in the company of people who are diametrically opposite of us. We believe wholeheartedly that our happiness lies in their hands, which creates the most tragic cycle of any kind of relationship.

If you stopped to think how finite your life is in terms of time, you would suddenly realize you don't want to waste it on people who don't enrich you and who, in fact, deplete you.

When I look back, my happiest memories are of when I was true to myself, even when it meant being judged by many at work or among friends and family. There is a sense of pride for standing up for what I believe. In fact, the times I have been most miserable is when I have found myself compromising on my respect, values and my belief system.

Surrounding yourself with the right people and making the right choices, as hard as they may be, is important for a healthy person, but imperative for a person living with a condition like Ulcerative Colitis. When you're with people who are wrong for you, you'll feel depleted, demoralized and stressed. The opposite is true when you are with those who love, support and celebrate you for who you are.

This is why the "right" person or the "right" choice should always be considered in context. There are people who may be toxic for us, but life experiences tell us that there are no absolutes and therefore, someone may be wrong for us but right for someone else. I would go as far as to say there are people and choices that are right for you and others that are simply not. I don't think I have ever regretted any choice I have made in life. Each one has taught me something and I am today the person I am because of those I met on the way and everything that I have experienced. It is this experience that has made me more discerning. I would rather spend my time today with those who validate my uniqueness as a human being, who take delight in what I bring to them, who take an interest in me; people who offer something to me, whether it's their wisdom, understanding or companionship.

But before I arrived at this understanding, I had to understand who the right people were for me. I learned that right doesn't mean chosen or better, it simply means those who are a comfortable and healthy fit for me. I found that I was happier when I was with people who I like, appreciate and respect and who have the same respect for me. I also realize that these are people I didn't "settle" for. I genuinely adore them; it wouldn't have been right if I had had to make a compromise to have them in my life.

This doesn't mean I am suggesting that we should only hang out with people who nod along to everything because they are afraid to voice their own opinions. Instead, I am talking of being among those who celebrate our good qualities and who are gentle but unafraid to tell us when we are making a bad choice or behaving out of character.

Being discerning also doesn't mean you put out a red velvet rope and decide to exclude all those who you think are wrong for you. I look at it like changing my diet to a healthy one. I know I have a finite appetite, so instead of telling myself not to eat deep fried and sugary things, I'd tell myself to eat more salads and fresh fruit. When I focus on what is healthy, I have less room for the unhealthy.

Being around people who are positive, happy and supportive helps me to be the same. It doesn't mean I have to be effervescent, but it does imply that I don't feel negated and stressed by them.

To make good use of a cliché: In the real world, we know that we can't be in a bubble with only those who are right for us. Discernment teaches you to prioritize people in your life. There may be people in your life who don't support you but may play a certain important role in your life. Well, they shouldn't simply be at the center of your life.

When I think of my world, I think of raindrops that fall on the surface of a pond and make little ripples. Discernment leads you to keep those who you care for and who genuinely care for you at the very center of your life's circle.

As you move outward, the rings include those who increasingly contribute less to your happiness and hold a lower position in your support structure. For most patients of chronic ailments like Ulcerative Colitis, our friends and family form one of the most critical support structures. It is therefore important to make choices that help us rather than make things worse for us.

I don't believe that the "right" people for me are of a certain personality, or have specific likes, dislikes or characteristics. It is more about finding resonance in each other, and the person I am when I'm with them.

Finding people who are right for you is not hugely different than finding the diet and lifestyle that is right for you. You try some things, you learn that they do you more harm than good, you move to those that do you good instead. It's about finding what your body, mind and spirit is comfortable with.

<u>When do you know it's right?</u>

When we are children, we have no shortage of "best friends." But as we get older, it gets harder to find genuine friendships, perhaps because the nature of friendship changes and hopefully, because we become more discerning. While there may not be a common characteristic or a share of likes and dislikes, there is a certain nature of a relationship that helps determine whether a person is right for you.

The right person is emotionally supportive and not unnecessarily critical of you. He or she listens to you thoughtfully and responds, rather than reacts, to what you've said.

One of the simplest ways to find out who really cares for you is when distance and time don't matter. When you're in a jam, you can call them - even at the last minute. Good friends inspire this confidence and reassurance. Even if you didn't meet until later in life, when you finally do, it feels just as it always did.

Good friends go out of their way for people they care about. They are thoughtful and perceptive. Being able to see someone else's needs and doing what you can to fulfill those needs deepens and strengthens a friendship. Our best friends do things for us that no one else would think of.

They are accepting of our flaws; when we are not at our best, they understand rather than complain. On my bad days with UC, friends of mine who care deeply and understand, ask me if they can help in any way or if I would prefer being by myself. Knowing that I have people I can trust reassures me that I have someone I can count on and who has my back.

I once read on a poster in a greeting card store: "Friends are therapists you can drink with." A great friendship is therapeutic; however, it isn't the same as having a drinking buddy. Sometimes we need a shoulder to cry on or a sympathetic ear, and having a friend you feel comfortable enough to share your deeper thoughts or emotions which is a wonderful gift.

On the flip side, it's important to recognize those who bring a bad energy around you. Sometimes you are only truly aware of the bad energy someone is bringing into your life when you're almost drowning in a pool of troubles by yourself; their adding on to it just raises a red flag in your mind. Generally, I've come to realize that there are some basic things that tell me when I'm with a person who isn't good for me.

Good friends make me feel energized and full of good ideas. They are not only comfortable with who I am they make me feel comfortable with myself as well. People who aren't right for me do exactly the opposite. I feel drained, defensive and unsettled. I also find that I am a much better person when I'm with good friends. These are healthy relationships and they promote a sense of well-being, not only around me but within me. As someone who suffers from UC, I know right away that friends who only have one way of socializing, namely drinking, eating junk food, talking negatively about other people or being extremely focused on wealth or status, aren't right for me. When I'm with them, I will either find myself getting sucked into such conversations and behavior or feel the negativity seep into my cells. In either situation, by the end of the evening I would feel worse about my world than at the start of the evening.

Dealing with those who drain you

People who drain our positive energy are always around us. We may find them at work or in our social life, but discerning and prioritizing the amount of importance and energy we pay them is key to learning how to manage them.

There are people who suck all the positive energy out of us to fuel their deep thirst for negativity. While they thrive on it, they leave us feeling exhausted and unhappy. They enjoy pointing out our inadequacies and love to remind us of our flaws. They like to prey on us when we're most vulnerable and take every opportunity to chip away at our self-confidence.

Often these are people who are intrusive, have a poor sense of boundaries, always have exaggerated reactions, are overly critical, complain about everything in their lives, are unable to take responsibility, are argumentative or demanding and many other such behavioral issues. Deep down, these are insecure, unhappy folks who have discovered they feel better about themselves when others feel worse.

The important thing I've learned is not to take their monkey onto my back – in other words, don't allow their problems to become yours. And the first step towards that is recognizing a potentially unhealthy influence in your life when you see one.

The negative nature of a person is not always apparent at first. I can say this from a very deep personal experience of my marriage and a later relationship. At first, their quirkiness may intrigue you; their stories may leave you wanting to hear more;

they may appear charming or their strife in life may make you sympathetic towards them. Soon, however, you begin to realize something is wrong. Don't ignore those feelings. Tune in to your gut. Pay close attention to your instincts and your physical reactions after your encounters. Our bodies know what is good and what is bad for us way before our mind is willing to admit it. If you find yourself experiencing muscle tension, loss of energy, headaches, irritability, a sense of disquiet or negativity, it is likely to be the impact of being with the wrong kind of person.

Once you've identified this, limit the amount of time you spend with such people. If you can't avoid them completely, such as in the case of family members or co-workers, set firm limits. For example, I use the following technique quite often to establish a boundary with people who tend to be very intrusive, or insist on offering highly dramatic tales or deluges of woes: I start my conversation with them with: "I only have a few minutes before I have to ....(either do something or go somewhere). And once this time is up, I politely disengage.

I've found this sends a subtle message to the other person that I'm not in a relationship where they can dump their negativity on me.

This is not to say I've become a cold and selfish person. I've just made it clear that I'm not going to invest myself in endless complaints or gossip. In fact, freeing myself from negativity allows me to focus on friends who do have genuine concerns and who I can actually help.

At the end of the day, I know no matter how much I might like to think or want to help, I will never be able to fix things for chronically negative people. They will either resist my help or invent new problems.

In such instances, I've found the best strategy is to protect myself by setting clear and firm boundaries. For example, I once told a friend who was perpetually unhappy with everything in her life and would actually compete with me in who was worse off, "I'm confident you'll find the right solution on your own," and excused myself. I don't believe in being rude, even to those who may be having a negative impact on me. But I do believe that being firm but empathetic helps in the long run.

I've realized that the power a person wields over you is given to them by you. There are people who will squeeze all the good energy out of you if you let them.

Finding the right people

Sometimes, when you're down and out and all you find are negative people around you, it feels like you have to settle; that there is no such thing as a "right" person. But I discovered a little secret, as I started to change the pattern in which I interacted with the world, I began to find more good friends than wrong ones. In order to attract the right people, we also have to put our own house in order. We have to be good friends ourselves, comfortable with our flaws, personalities and needs.

Over the years, through coming to terms with my chronic ailment and how it has changed my life, I have also learned to enjoy my own company. A yoga teacher once told me, we expect others in the world to live with us happily, but ironically we are often not comfortable living with ourselves.

It helps to be socially participatory rather than leave everything up to serendipity. I once dug into my old phonebook to find friends I had lost touch with over the years but who I remembered to be essentially positive people.

Another way is to create opportunities and spaces where you're likely to meet a greater number and variety of people. Striking a balance is essential because if your time and energy is misspent on the wrong relationships or too many activities, you'll end up neglecting your good relationships and in a self-defeating cycle of fleeting friendships and superficial relationships that may be thrilling in the short run but meaningless in the long run.

Sometimes, we have to start afresh. When you clean out and de-clutter your closet, you have to go out shopping for a new wardrobe. This period also gives you the perfect opportunity to spend time on your own.

For me, the appreciation of solitude started with enjoying the sense of freedom it came with it. There were no pressures to go out or appear cheerful even at times when I wasn't. Also, I realized when you enjoy your own company, you don't need others for the sake of filling a gap but because you genuinely enjoy spending time with them. You don't enter relationships out of a fear of being alone, but because they bring something of value to you.

Besides, when you're desperate for the company of others, you will most likely be less authentic and more focused on pleasing them; hungry for approval rather than letting people know the real you.

One of the ways I spend quality time with myself is when I go for a walk or when I sometimes travel on my own. The goal is to get to the point where you achieve a healthy balance between staying in by yourself and going out with friends and being equally happy doing both.

Joining groups centered on faith, community or charity work or hobbies is very helpful to finding others who share a common value or love for something.

A shared passion is the most effective component in building positive and lasting relationships. I've also found that one of the best investments I have made in myself is to take a genuine interest in my friends. Love and kindness begets love and kindness.

CHAPTER 11

FAMILY, FRIENDS, & SUPPORT STRUCTURE

I must admit that even today I find it difficult to discuss my condition with friends, family or others. It is has been a lonely battle I have fought for so long that it is too close to home to share easily. Perhaps writing this book is partly a process of catharsis and an attempt to be free from this inability to talk about the disease. To some extent, however, the highly private and embarrassing nature of this disease prevents our families and friends from truly understanding what we go through and from being there for us in a constructive way.

Resources and materials on Ulcerative Colitis in the public domain are often directed to the patient and how he or she can cope with the disease and miss out on explaining the role that partners, family and friends play in support and care giving.

Hence this is a chapter I'd like to address to all those who may be reading this book because they have someone they care deeply for who suffers from Ulcerative Colitis.

For people closest to a patient of UC, the story begins only once you truly know what is happening to the person physically, emotionally and mentally. I remember at first I didn't talk to anyone about my diagnosis. I was married at the time, and although my husband somewhat understood the physical aspects of the disease, he had no idea of the ramifications of the disease. My mother very quickly knew that something was wrong with me. My dramatic loss of weight was the first tip-off; then my lack of energy and socializing were a giveaway to my friends. Not to mention the fact that I wasn't eating or drinking very much. But overall, I found it extremely difficult to talk about it. I made my excuses and retreated from the rest of the world for the roughest part of my battle with the disease. I'm aware that the reason I found myself alone through the darkest of times was partly because I had decided to exclude world, and partly because those close to me didn't truly understand how they could be there for me.

For every patient of Ulcerative Colitis, I believe, the decision to share or not is personal – he or she decides when they are ready to talk about their health. But as a friend, partner or family member, you have to demonstrate patience and, depending on how close or involved you are in their care, your learning curve about the disease has to be as sharp as the person suffering from it.

When your loved one is sick, the desire to make her or him feel better can be overwhelming, and so can be the helplessness you feel during one of their flare-ups. You may not always be able to do a great deal, but a good place to start is to reduce your partner's stress and support him or her in the lifestyle changes that come with having Ulcerative Colitis.

A study conducted in 1988 showed researchers the impact of the diagnosis of a serious or chronic illness on the family of the person suffering from it. The study found that there are three major and immediate aspects. The person diagnosed with the ailment experiences (a) new stressors; (b) new resources; and then (c) the person assigns meaning to the crisis. Stressors can include a whole new set of demands on them which could be physical, emotional and mental. To help balance out these new stressors, the person starts to rely on a certain support system. This is where friends and family enter the picture – they become the resource the person can count on. The search for meaning is a journey that the person undertakes mostly on his or her own. The study determined that in the long run, all three aspects (stressors, resources and meaning) join together to determine if the person will adapt positively or negatively to this new reality. For your part in the outcome, being aware of the following could be quite useful.

Food and society

For example, if it's your partner who has UC, become conscious of the food choices you can make as a couple. Whether you go grocery shopping or eat out, it may be hard for your partner to see you being able to eat anything you want, while he or she may dread every meal not knowing how it will impact her.

You can support your partner by cooking healthy meals that you can enjoy together. Take note of things that don't agree with him or her, paying even greater attention to foods that help the person.

Socializing often takes a big hit for a UC patient during flare-ups or uncertain periods. Another big way to help your loved one is to be supportive and not pressure her or him during these periods. When you do go out with friends and family, know that people may not always understand why your partner refuses to have dessert or a glass of wine. If your partner is finding it hard to extricate himself from the situation politely or the hosts are pressuring him too much, step in and speak up for your partner. If your partner is uncomfortable sharing information about his health, simply say something like, "John has a lot of food allergies, so he has to be careful about what he eats."

When you both go out, remember food is not the only point of concern for a UC patient. It would be a huge help to your partner if you keep in mind whether the toilets are clean where you are going, and to know if they are private and accessible. Your partner will be able to enjoy the evening far better when she or he knows that there is a clean restroom close to him or her just in case there's a need to go.

The learning curve

Knowledge is one of the key weapons in any battle, and this is truer when it comes to health issues. If your partner was recently diagnosed with Ulcerative Colitis, or if you just found out about your loved one's condition, a good place to start is reading up on the subject. There are ample resources online as well as in public libraries that will make you an informed caregiver. The more educated you are on the nature of the disease and how symptoms come and go, the more empathetic you can be for your loved one. Being knowledgeable about Ulcerative Colitis can also allow you to speak more freely about medication side effects that may be affecting your loved one or changes in their symptoms that you may notice. These discussions can reassure your loved one and help him or her to better deal with the symptoms and feel more in control of the disease.

Always remember that Ulcerative Colitis is very individualized, and often what may work or not work for one person may be completely different for another person. So it's good to keep talking with your partner. Keeping the lines of communication open between your partner and you is critical; otherwise the severity of symptoms may go unchecked. Especially because a person suffering UC often needs a little encouragement and understanding in order to open up about their feelings or symptoms.

If it is a friend who has the ailment, increasing your knowledge about UC helps in planning outings; your friend will be more willing to go out with someone who understands and is supportive than someone who may be tactless or intrusive. Also, you'll know when not to pressure her too much into going out or doing something you know she can't do or doesn't feel comfortable with.

<u>Plan and prepare</u>

When you have a partner, family member or friend who suffers from Ulcerative Colitis, you quickly learn that plans can get cancelled suddenly and you have to be prepared. Travelling, in particular, can be a complicated endeavor. However, you can dissolve some of your own and your partner's anxieties by planning ahead and preparing yourself for any outcome. When booking seats on airlines or buses, ask for seats closest to the bathroom. When choosing a destination, food, hygiene and availability of clean toilets should be considered.

Be prepared for your partner's body to change. Not only does having UC result in dramatic loss of weight, but medications like steroids impact the way your partner looks. I can say from firsthand experience that taking steroids may be necessary but also one of the harshest treatments for your body to endure. I remember feeling horrible because of severe mood swings, weight gain from water retention, sleeplessness and puffiness in the face. I can tell you during this time, it's really important to pay your partner compliments and being appreciative of him or her. Even small gestures of love and thoughtfulness will bring them happiness. Consistent emotional support is extremely important because both of you have your individual pressures and vulnerabilities.

When you are a partner or close family member, while you are looking after and supporting the person with UC, you also have to remember to look after yourself as well. You can only be a good caregiver and partner when you yourself are in a good state of emotional and physical health.

In fact, sometimes when you are a caregiver it can be very easy to neglect yourself. The emotional impact of caring for someone with Ulcerative Colitis can be highly stressful. You may be asked to be actively involved in the patient's life in ways that are unfamiliar and uncomfortable. Acknowledging this fact is important both for you and your loved one. For you to be a supportive caregiver, it is essential that you take care of yourself, get enough rest and exercise and eat a well-balanced diet. If your partner is unable to go out for long periods of time, make sure you don't bring your own social life to a complete standstill. As much as your partner may need a support structure of friends and family, you need one too.

How a family copes

In the last ten years, I've read many accounts of men and women who suffer from Ulcerative Colitis and about how the dynamics of this disease impacts not just one individual, but the family as a whole. It poses challenges to parenting as well as to fulfilling other responsibilities a person carries in a family. Whether it's attending to children, elders in the family or even carrying out the duties of a partner.

And as members of a family, you may have a host of feelings, including neglect, resentment and anger towards the patient for disrupting your life and making demands on you. The reverse happens, too. You may have to bear the brunt of being the person who is suffering from UC and who feels a myriad of strong emotions: frustration, envy of others who can enjoy life and guilt for putting their loved ones through an ordeal, too.

Then there are uncertainties – will the family be able to take that holiday or go hiking on the weekend?

I think some of the principles that apply to the person with Ulcerative Colitis apply to a family as well. The same principles will help in easing the anxieties and minimizing disappointment. For example, the reality of the situation is that there is a loved one in the family who suffers from this condition, and that they may have an unannounced flare-up that could put a damper on any plan. It is therefore better to manage the depth of your own expectations than to experience a crushing disappointment.

Discuss within the family whether it will be okay for some members of the family to take a holiday sometimes without having to plan for everyone to always go together. Going away, even for a short break, is important for everyone involved because it will reduce some of the stress of coping with the disease. I would say the same to a patient of UC as well: for the family's health, and in some way to reduce your own guilt, it's a good idea to explain that you will be absolutely fine with them taking a holiday on their own every now and then, especially activities they may enjoy but may be difficult for you to take on.

Honesty along with creativity can help children in the family deal with disappointments. I recently read a very valuable suggestion for a parent with UC. When there are very young children involved who may not understand the disease or that a parent is sick and may be unable to go to the park or engage in a planned activity, it is a good idea to explain that there's something going on in your body, and instead suggest an indoor activity like baking or crafts, or simply watching a movie together. This way you still spend quality time together and engage in something together.

Handling unexpected flare-ups and complications

An Ulcerative Colitis flare-up sometimes comes on all of a sudden and symptoms can be severe stomach cramps, diarrhea that may have blood, or abdominal pain. As a caregiver, you sometimes need to help your partner decide whether it is one that merits a trip to the emergency room. There are some situations, however, when a visit to the hospital is imperative and you make a call to his or her doctor. When the person has a fast heart rate, high fever and more than ten bowel movements a day with lots of blood, it's time to seek immediate medical attention.

There are also certain complications like a toxic mega colon. This is a potentially life-threatening complication of Ulcerative Colitis. The large intestines become paralyzed, stop working and get hugely inflamed – so much so that you would see a visibly distended abdomen. The patient may have increasingly worsening abdominal pain, tenderness in the region, high fever, dehydration and a sudden decrease in the number of bowel movements. If this complication is not treated, the intestine can get perforated leading to infection and even death.

This brings me to another set of complications related to Ulcerative Colitis: Perforated Bowel and Hemorrhaging Perforated Bowel. These complications may lead to heavy rectal bleeding or hemorrhaging. Perforation not only occurs as a result of toxic mega colon, but can also be caused by infection, certain medications, or long-term ulcers in the colon. The reason this complication needs to be addressed immediately is because perforation can lead the intestinal bacteria to travel to the rest of the body, causing a massive infection and possibly even death.

As a caregiver, you need to keep a checklist and ask your partner if he or she saw a dramatic increase in the amount of blood in their stool.

Things you shouldn't say

In the last ten years, I've come across three main types of people in the context of my condition: those who are genuinely caring, helpful and don't have an intrusive manner; those who have a ton of good intentions, but believe they know much better about you and your life than you do; and those who are simply uncaring, tactless and approach life with negative energy. All of the above have never suffered from Ulcerative Colitis and while their level of comprehension may vary greatly, none truly understand the illness completely. I've heard many things that today I feel no patient of Ulcerative Colitis should ever hear. So, as those who don't have the disease but may interact with friends or family who do, I must tell you, there are some things you should never say.

No supermodel jokes or size zero envy

People with UC often lose weight dramatically and sometimes they may look puffy due to the steroids they are prescribed. As patients, we are painfully aware of how our appearance has changed. We don't need someone else to confirm it or remark on it. And it's even more hurtful, when friends make statements like, "Oh how I wish I was as thin as you!" I don't think anyone who suffers from UC would ever wish this kind of weight-loss upon a friend.

Don't discount the illness

Don't play the illness down just because you may not be able to cope with its seriousness. I once heard someone tell me, "You don't look sick." Instead of saying "You don't look sick" you can pay a genuine compliment like "You look lovely today."

It's not a grief competition

There are some people who must outdo everyone else...even when it comes to serious situations like ill health. I once heard someone tell me, "Oh this is nothing. I had a tumor on my leg five years ago and had to get it operated on!" I don't think anyone wants to hear that they don't have it as bad as someone else. Each person's troubles are large and significant to them.

Don't fake empathy

You don't have to empathize with someone in order to show your support. Just knowing they can count on you for support and understanding is enough. Some years ago, a friend came up to me and said, "I know what you're going through. I had a stomach infection once and it was horrible."

This is a life-long illness that requires constant maintenance, long periods of hospitalization, severe medication and involves a great deal of pain. Instead of faking empathy, offer real, practical support by asking if there's anything you can help them with when they are sick.

Don't overdo concern

If you are out with a friend who has UC and needs to go to the toilet often, you don't have to ask them about how things are on every return trip they make to the toilet. For him or her, it can be an added stress to manage a hyper-anxious friend. Don't jump or remark every time you hear your friend's stomach rumble or make a noise either.

<u>Don't say, "Eat more fiber"</u>

Fiber really is the last thing your friend should be eating. It may be applicable to people with a case of loose motions, but it isn't applicable to people with inflammatory bowel diseases. In fact, fiber can cause more pressure on her digestive system than resolve any issue. I cannot stress this enough that each person who suffers from Ulcerative Colitis has to figure out what works and what doesn't for his or her gut through a long process of trial and error. There is no flat rule that applies to all. And fiber definitely isn't the magic cure that escaped your friend and her doctor's notice.

The same goes for insisting that your friend have that glass of wine or take just one bite of that cheeseburger. Understand the reality: your friend may love cheeseburgers, but today even a bite may send her into a spell of diarrhea and pain. So it's already hard for her to resist, don't make it worse.

A chronic illness is not easy on the person suffering it, or on those around him or her. It's better for everyone involved to remain sensitive, genuine and reassuring.

THE END